the complete illustrated guide to

VITAMINS AND
MINERALS

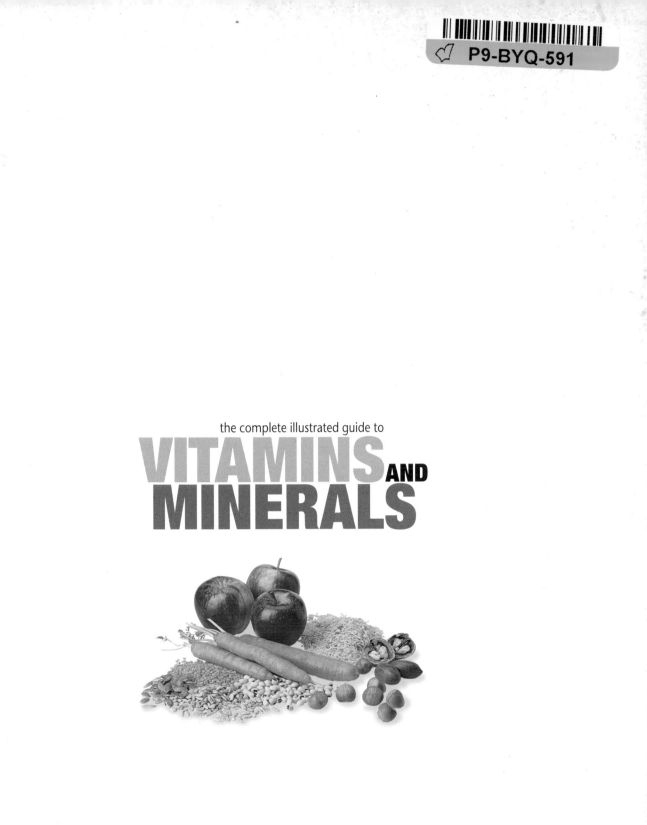

the complete illustrated guide to

VITAMINS AND MINERALS

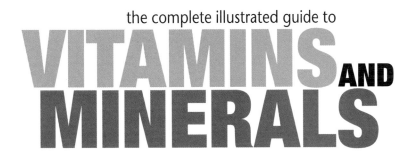

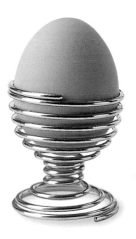

DENISE MORTIMORE

ELEMENT

Element
An Imprint of HarperCollins*Publishers*
77–85 Fulham Palace Road
Hammersmith, London W6 8JB

First published in Great Britain in 2001 by
Element

10 9 8 7 6 5 4 3 2 1

A catalogue record for this book
is available from the British Library

ISBN 0007122462

Printed and bound in Great Britain by
Butler & Tanner, Frome and London
Reprographics in Singapore by
Bright Arts Graphic (Pte) Ltd

This book was designed, and produced by
THE BRIDGEWATER BOOK COMPANY

EDITORIAL DIRECTOR Fiona Biggs
DESIGN DIRECTOR Terry Jeavons
ART DIRECTOR Michael Whitehead
DESIGNER Jane Lanaway
PROJECT EDITOR Sarah Bragginton
PICTURE RESEARCHER Liz Moore
PHOTOGRAPHER Ian Parsons

Acknowledgements

The publishers wish to thank the
following for use of library pictures:

Associated Press: 17t; Cephas: 113l, 155; Bruce Coleman
Collection: 121l; Corbis UK Ltd: 75; Getty Stone: 13t, 22b,
36bl, 51t, 64l, 68–9t, 72, 82t, 99b, 103t, 106b, 110–11b,
118t, 129t, 132b, 143t, 144–5b, 146–7t, 150c, 163b, 164c,
170–1b, 177, 182; Hutchison Library: 69br;
Image Bank: 45, 66b; Images Colour Library: 176, 183;
Science Photo Library: 24tl, 30t, 33t, 38–39b, 51br, 52b, 54,
55t, 70r, 137br, 138–9, 160t, 165b, 173, 180; Stock Market:
141t; Superstock: 117, 124–5b
(t=top, b=bottom, l=left, r=right, c=centre)

The publishers would also like to thank Indexing Specialists
for compiling the index in this book.

CONTENTS

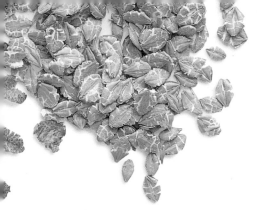

PART FOUR OPTIMIZING YOUR DIET 130

PART FIVE PROBLEM SOLVING 152

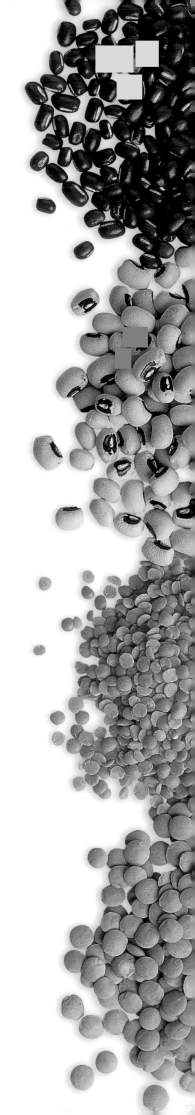

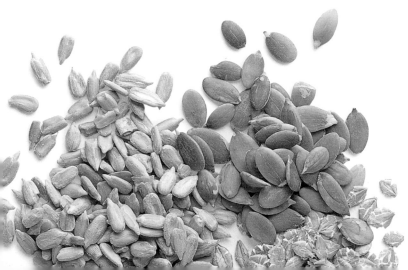

HOW TO USE THIS BOOK

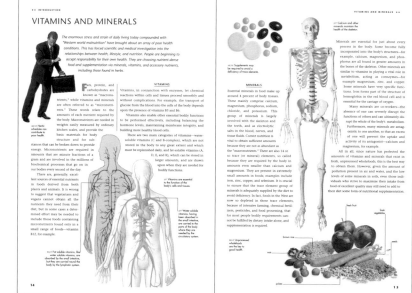

*This book comprises five main sections. **Part One: Introduction** details the importance of eating well and introduces vitamins and minerals and their recommended daily amounts. **Part Two: The Vitamins** lists all the known vitamins and their functions, lists the foods that they significantly occur in, details the recommended daily amount, and describes deficiency and overdose symptoms. **Part Three: The Minerals** lists all the main minerals and their functions, lists the foods that they significantly occur in, details the recommended daily amount, and describes deficiency and overdose symptoms. **Part Four: Optimizing your Diet** shows you how to improve your health and well-being through making changes to what you eat and with the judicious use of vitamin and mineral supplements, while **Part Five: Problem Solving** details problems with specific body systems and parts, and shows how certain supplements can help keep these healthy and in the best condition possible.*

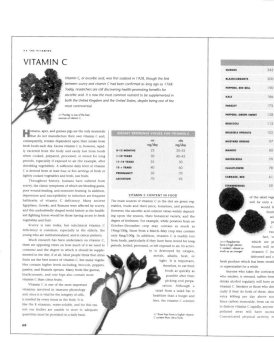

Part One: Introduction describes the importance of eating well and how vitamins and minerals work. How to take supplements safely is also discussed.

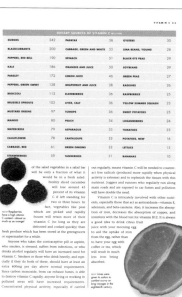

Part Two: The Vitamins lists all the known vitamins, what they are, what the recommended daily amount is, and what foods they occur in.

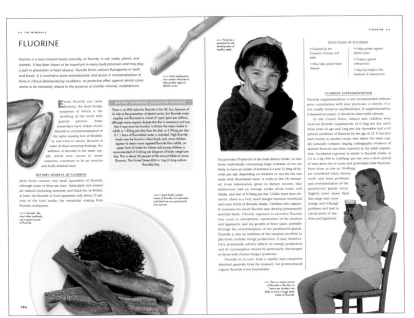

Part Three: The Minerals lists all the known minerals, what they are, how they should be taken, the recommended daily amount, and what foods they occur in.

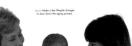

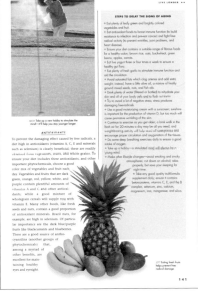

Part Four: Optimizing your Diet shows you how to increase your energy levels, improve your immune system, and fight infection through diet and proper supplement use.

Part Five: Problem Solving details specific illnesses and diseases that affect the main systems of the body and how these can be treated with nutritional supplements and diet.

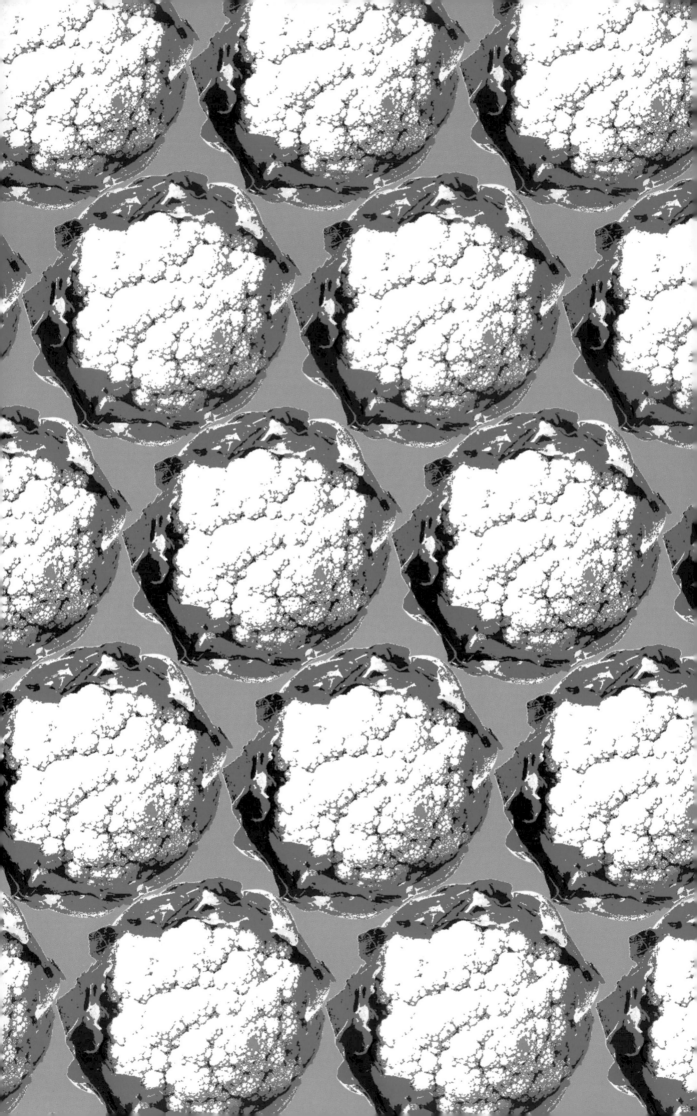

PART ONE

INTRODUCTION

Food is far more than just fuel. It has always been clear that food has a medicinal effect and that a varied diet, rich in natural ingredients, is a prerequisite for good health. Understanding our own bodies is the fundamental basis of both preventive healthcare and treatment—and understanding what we put in our bodies is even more important. It is vital that we realize that diet has an enormous impact on our physical and mental health, and that the food we eat has both therapeutic and preventive benefits. We must begin to recognize the fact that our health problems may be caused by the foods we are, or are not, eating—after all, it's in our own hands.

INTRODUCTION

Choosing what we eat is one of the simplest and most effective ways to influence our health. Various factors affect our choice—time, lifestyle, even our emotions. We often feel the need to eat quickly, to have something fatty, sugary, and comforting. Soon we are feeling either worse or are craving more comfort food. Fresh food is often an afterthought. But as our knowledge of the positive power of good food and its nutrients grows, eating will become a pleasurable act during which the body is given its vital nourishment. Nutritional supplements, and up-to-date information about them, are also important.

RIGHT Snacking on fruit is both tasty and healthy.

During our lifetime, we may go through several changes in our eating practices—many people take the decision to become vegetarian, for example. Healthy living includes a flexible approach to our growth and needs, since what we eat represents more than simply ingesting nutrients—it is an expression of how we feel about ourselves. The basic nutrients essential for life are available in a whole range of different foods, enabling meat-eaters, vegetarians, and vegans to choose from a range of high-vitality foods to maximize the intake of these essential substances.

The human body has fundamental requirements—fats, proteins, carbohydrates, energy, water, and oxygen. On top of these, it needs some 40 different vitamins, minerals, essential amino acids, and essential fatty acids

RIGHT The human body needs a combination of elements to maintain optimum health.

to remain healthy. A deficiency in any of the nutrients will result in anything from mild to chronic ill health. Single nutrient deficiencies tend to be rare, but multiple deficiencies often occur, particularly in people who are already suffering from another illness.

Multiple mild, subclinical deficiencies are common in individuals who eat a typical Western diet, characterized by its many excesses and its lack of essential nutrients. We are "overfed and undernourished." Furthermore, nutrient-deficient food and diets that include large and frequent amounts of common allergens (wheat, yeast, milk, eggs, citrus, and alcohol) can impair digestion, irritate the gut lining, and lead to a range of food intolerances in susceptible individuals. In addition to this, don't forget environmental pollutants, overuse of antibiotics and other drugs, and drinking alcohol to excess—all of these impair the body's ability to absorb and assimilate nutrients. When combined these different factors may eventually lead to degenerative disease and chronic ill health.

RIGHT Some of the most commonly used foods can cause allergies in susceptible individuals.

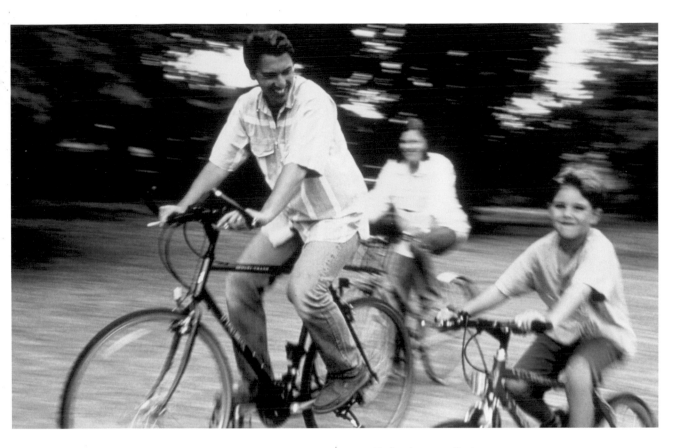

ABOVE **Cycling is an excellent way for the whole family to exercise in the fresh air.**

AMOUNTS OF INDIVIDUAL NUTRIENTS

International units (IU) are related to the activity of vitamins A, D, and E. Many supplements contain these vitamins in IU amounts, some will be in weights and some will give both. All other vitamins and minerals are given as weight. All food lists are given in amounts that equate to the units used for RDAs or RNIs.

1 IU vitamin A = 0.3mcg

1 IU vitamin D = 0.025mcg

1 IU vitamin E = 0.7mg, as D-alpha tocopherol

microgram = mcg

milligram (1,000mcg) = mg

gram (1,000mg) = g

In order to regain a feeling of complete physical and mental well-being, we need to learn more about the essential vitamins and minerals.

Governments around the world have provided guidelines for how much of the major vitamins and minerals we need in our diets. The United States and mainland Europe use the RDA (recommended dietary allowance/ recommended daily allowance/recommended daily amount), which applies to healthy individuals with a good balanced diet. The United Kingdom uses RDAs and RNIs (reference nutrient intake) that relate to an amount that should be sufficient for 97 percent of the people in any one group. Here we will use the United States RDA and the UK RNI. These levels are, however, for "adequate" intake and do not reflect new thinking for optimal health and longevity. They are not therapeutic levels and they do not take into account the varying needs of the population with regard to state of health, activity, or lifestyle. Supplements available for self-prescription often contain many times the RDA or RNI levels and so are moderately therapeutic. If, however, you plan to take large doses of vitamins and minerals, contact your practitioner for advice beforehand.

This book will provide you with a concise, up-to-date review of all the vitamins and minerals currently regarded by the scientific and medical professions to be important to good health. You will find details of daily requirements for each nutrient and examples of which foods are likely to supply them in the highest and most accessible amounts. In addition, information on nutrient functions, deficiency symptoms, and nutritional supplementation is provided for each vitamin and mineral.

RIGHT **Even the healthiest diet can sometimes benefit from supplements.**

VITAMINS AND MINERALS

The enormous stress and strain of daily living today compounded with "Western world malnutrition" have brought about an array of poor health conditions. This has forced scientific and medical investigation into the relationships between health, lifestyle, and nutrition. People are beginning to accept responsibility for their own health. They are choosing nutrient-dense food and supplementation via minerals, vitamins, and accessory nutrients, including those found in herbs.

ABOVE Hectic schedules can contribute to poor health.

Fats, protein, and carbohydrates are known as "macronutrients," while vitamins and minerals are often referred to as "micronutrients." These words relate to the amounts of each nutrient required by the body. Macronutrients are needed in weights easily measured by ordinary kitchen scales, and provide the basic materials for body structure and for substances that can be broken down to provide energy. Micronutrients are required in amounts that are minute fractions of a gram and are involved in the millions of biochemical processes that go on in our bodies every second of the day.

There are, generally, excellent sources of essential nutrients in foods derived from both plants and animals. It is wrong to suggest that vegetarians and vegans cannot obtain all the nutrients they need from their diet, but in some cases a determined effort may be needed to include those foods containing micronutrients found only in a small range of foods—vitamin B12, for example.

RIGHT Fat-soluble vitamins, like water soluble vitamins, are absorbed by the small intestine, but they are carried round the body by the lymphatic system.

VITAMINS

Vitamins, in conjunction with enzymes, let chemical reactions within cells and tissues proceed smoothly and without complications. For example, the transport of glucose from the blood into the cells of the body depends upon the presence of vitamins B3 and B6.

Vitamins also enable other essential bodily functions to be performed effectively, including balancing the hormone levels, maintaining membrane integrity, and building more healthy blood cells.

There are two main categories of vitamins—water-soluble vitamins (C and B-complex), which are not stored in the body to any great extent and which must be replenished daily, and fat-soluble vitamins (A, D, E, and K), which can be stored in larger amounts, and are drawn upon when they are needed for bodily functions.

LEFT Vitamins are essential to the function of the body's cells and tissues.

LEFT Water soluble vitamins, having been absorbed in the small intestine, are carried to the parts of the body where they are needed by the circulatory system.

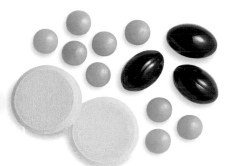

ABOVE Supplements may be required to avoid a deficiency of trace elements.

LEFT Calcium and other minerals maintain the health of the skeleton.

MINERALS

Essential minerals in food make up around 4 percent of body tissues. These mainly comprise calcium, magnesium, phosphorus, sodium, chloride, and potassium. This group of minerals is largely involved with the skeleton and the teeth, and as electrolytic salts in the blood, nerves, and tissue fluids. Correct nutrition is vital to obtain sufficient amounts because they are not as abundant as the "macronutrients." There are also 14 or so trace (or mineral) elements, so called because they are required by the body in amounts even smaller than calcium and magnesium. They are present in extremely small amounts in foods; examples include iron, zinc, copper, and selenium. It is crucial to ensure that the trace element group of minerals is adequately supplied by the diet to avoid deficiency. In fact, foods in the West are now so depleted in these trace elements, because of intensive farming, chemical fertilizers, pesticides, and food processing, that for most people bodily requirements cannot be fulfilled by dietary intake alone, and supplementation is required.

Minerals are essential for just about every process in the body. Some become fully incorporated into the body's structures—for example, calcium, magnesium, and phosphorus are all found in greater amounts in the bones of the skeleton. Other minerals are similar to vitamins in playing a vital role in metabolism, acting as coenzymes—for example magnesium, zinc, and copper. Some minerals have very specific functions. Iron forms part of the structure of hemoglobin in the red blood cell and is essential for the carriage of oxygen.

Many minerals are co-workers—the absence of one can severely disrupt the functions of others and can ultimately disrupt the whole of the body's metabolism. Furthermore, many minerals are antagonistic to one another, so that an excess of one will prevent the uptake and activity of its antagonist—calcium and magnesium, for example.

All in all, since nature has perfected the amounts of vitamins and minerals that exist in fresh, unprocessed wholefoods, this is the best way to obtain them. However, given the amount of pollution present in air and water, and the low levels of some minerals in soils, even those individuals who strive to maximize their intake from food of excellent quality may still need to add to their diet some form of nutritional supplementation.

RIGHT Unprocessed wholefoods are the key to good health.

fresh fruit

fresh vegetables

brown rice

seeds

nuts

pulses

MODERN DIET AND ITS IMBALANCES

The typical diet in the western world provides far from adequate nutrition. It seems unbelievable that those of us who enjoy a standard of living unparalleled in history should include among our number many who are malnourished. This is often a reflection of the stressful lives we lead, in which there is little time for eating proper meals. Food is often eaten "on the hoof" and good nutrition is rarely a priority. We choose quick, high-carbohydrate, fatty, refined food and are much more guided by "mouth hunger" than real hunger. This "civilized" diet actually contributes to obesity, heart disease, cancer, digestive disorders, premature aging, diabetes, osteoporosis and many autoimmune diseases like arthritis.

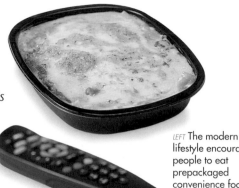

LEFT The modern lifestyle encourages people to eat prepackaged convenience foods and "TV dinners."

Many diseases would be prevented, or even cured, by proper nutrition and a healthier lifestyle. Although much money is spent on health care, degenerative diseases are still on the increase. The current high intake of saturated fat, refined carbohydrates and sugar, meat, and dairy products appears to be a major cause of cancer, heart disease, diabetes, and osteoporosis, since diets high in these foods are almost always extremely low in nutrient-dense food like vegetables, pulses, seeds, and fruit.

Modern large-scale food-processing—for example, the refining of flour—is detrimental to the nutritional quality of food. When flour is refined, dietary fiber, essential vitamins (particularly the B group), and minerals are removed. These are the very nutrients that are needed inside the body to turn starchy food, like flour, into energy.

Not only are essential nutrients being removed from food during processing, but in order to make food easier to transport, distribute, and prepare in the home, convenience foods have flooded on to the market. To make these "easy-to-cook," preservative-loaded foods look more colorful and appealing (since all their natural flavors and colors have been lost during the processing), artificial substances are added by the manufacturers. Many of these substances can be harmful to susceptible individuals. Furthermore, although we are assured by the controlling agencies that each food additive has undergone rigorous tests to ensure its safety, most present-day food additives

ABOVE A healthy diet should include unrefined foods such as whole grains and seeds.

have not been tested in groups (as they would appear in food) and, therefore, their synergistic (combined) effects are mostly unknown.

If this wasn't enough, much of the food we eat has been sprayed, injected, grown in chemically rich soil, or fed on unsuitable food. Additionally, we now find that the very basis of life—the DNA—is being tampered with. Genetically modified foods are creeping in all around us.

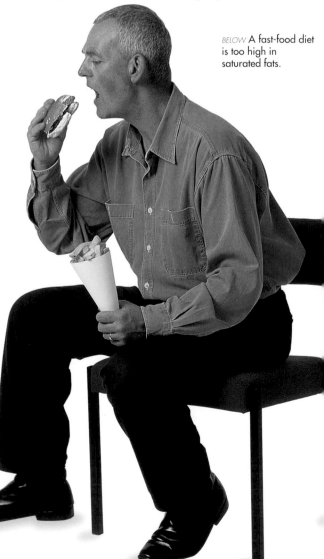

BELOW A fast-food diet is too high in saturated fats.

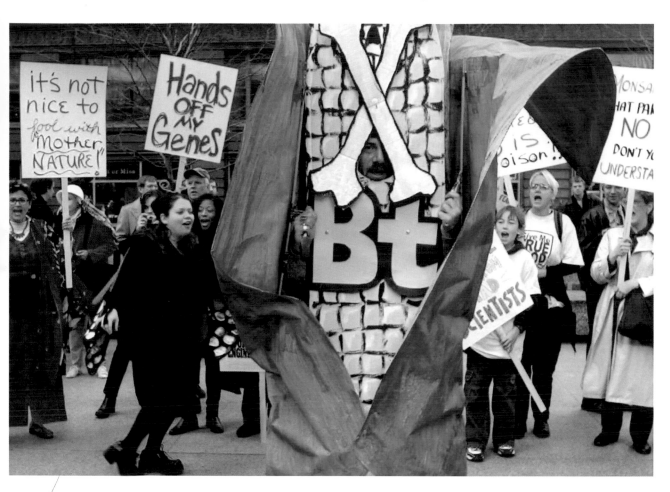

The long-term effects of all of these procedures on our health are yet to be investigated thoroughly. What is obvious is that the ability of our bodies to convert these non-food, abnormal, toxin-laden chemicals into safe substances that can be quickly eliminated by the liver and kidneys is becoming grossly impaired. The Western diet overfeeds and undernourishes. This is in contrast to some developing countries where there is often insufficient food of any kind to sustain a proper healthy life. True "under-nutrition" such as this is seldom found in Western countries except in sufferers of anorexia, bulimia, or other severe illnesses. What we do suffer from is malnutrition—"bad" nutrition.

Things are beginning to change, fortunately, and government agencies, educational establishments, and the media have managed to get the "low fat" message across. However, the additional problems of chemically adulterated, over-processed, nutrient-deficient food, are yet to be fully recognized. The general public appear to be making their stand on genetically modified foods, but if this "united voice" truly does want food that will nourish and strengthen our bodies in the way it is meant to, it also needs to reject the synthetic, chemical food we have been eating for the last two or three decades.

Nourishing a body back to health, unfortunately, is not simply a case of cutting out the fat, sugar, and chemicals, and providing standard amounts of essential

ABOVE **Demonstrators protest over genetically modified foods.**

nutrients while reducing the number of calories. We are, every one of us, unique and because of this require different amounts of nutrients depending on our age, present state of health, gender, occupation, and activity level. Additionally, any problems we may have in our digestive system, or any reduction in absorptive capacity will, similarly, lead to differing nutritional requirements. The next section will provide you with some information that is worth considering when trying to assess your own body and your individual nutritional needs.

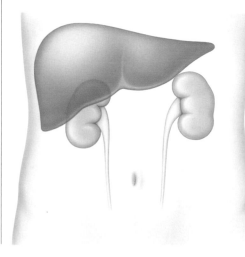

LEFT **Toxins are safely eliminated via the liver and kidneys. They also escape via the lungs and the skin.**

BIOCHEMICAL INDIVIDUALITY

RIGHT As we grow older, we need to increase our nutrient intake.

Everyone has their own optimum range of nutrient intake that determines whether or not a person remains healthy. Tables of nutritional requirements provide some guidance, but these can only give very general information. Our nutrient levels are influenced by many factors including gender, stage of growth, activity levels, age, state of general health, and degree of stress. Nutritional tables often give differing values for some of these factors but the additional information, given in this book, enables you to decide where you need to amend these intakes further.

GENDER

Nutrient requirements are different for males and females. A woman's nutritional requirements can vary throughout the menstrual cycle, especially if she is taking the contraceptive pill, and lack of certain nutrients may contribute to PMS, and other problems. Menstrual loss means that many women have iron requirements above those of men of the same age. Young adolescent males may need more zinc than a female of the same age since this is required for sperm production and generation of male hormones.

GROWTH

A growing body has a higher need for many nutrients. Protein, essential fatty acids, and certain minerals, such as zinc and iron, are required in greater amounts, in relation to body weight, by children at puberty than by adults.

PREGNANCY AND LACTATION

A pregnant or breastfeeding woman generally requires more nutrients. In particular, the need for folic acid and other vitamins and minerals is increased to ensure healthy development of the fetus, and calcium needs are increased during the breastfeeding period to ensure proper development of the child's skeleton.

LEFT Pregnancy requires a woman to take more nutrients, for example folic acid.

STATE OF GENERAL HEALTH

Many illnesses and diseases severely deplete resources of certain nutrients, particularly where there are digestive and absorption problems or where diarrhea is a symptom. Acute viral illnesses, such as the common cold or influenza, will increase the need for zinc, vitamin C, and other nutrients.

AGE

As we get older, we almost certainly will require greater amounts of certain essential nutrients, both to combat the wear and tear of an aging metabolism and digestive system and to counteract the nutrient-depleting effect of any medication. National tables do not reflect this and to complicate matters, calorific intake needs to be reduced as we age.

DIGESTIVE CAPABILITIES

A person whose digestion is inefficient is likely to have a higher requirement for nutrients. This may be caused by insufficient production of hydrochloric acid in the stomach or poor digestive enzyme production by the pancreas and other enzyme-secreting glands. Poor digestion is often the start of food sensitivity or food intolerance, leading to a still further increase in the requirements of essential nutrients.

RIGHT Poor digestion means more nutrients need to be taken.

RIGHT Smoking increases the need for some vitamins and minerals.

BELOW Tea and coffee can lead to poor absorption of some nutrients.

ABSORPTION

Several vital nutrients, including B vitamins, iron, and zinc, are poorly absorbed in the presence of mild stimulants such as tea and coffee. Inhibitor substances such as anti-iodine goiterogens in Brassicas, or phytates in cereals also interfere with absorption. Coffee, and tea, is better between meals rather than with them and thyroid sufferers should always cook Brassica vegetables to inactivate the goiterogens. Mineral-high foods and supplements are best taken at meals that do not contain cereals.

ASSIMILATION

Assimilation is the process by which nutrients are used by the body once they have been absorbed. Some people have metabolic faults. These may be as a result of genetic defect, food intolerance, nutritional deficiencies, food toxins, and environmental pollutants that prevent the body from efficiently utilizing the nutrients they have absorbed. For example, children are affected particularly badly by cadmium, found in tobacco smoke and lead from petrol fumes. These pollutants prevent the assimilation of nutrients within the body and may be a cause of childhood hyperactivity and attention deficit disorders.

PSYCHOLOGICAL AND EMOTIONAL STRESS

Stress increases the requirements of certain nutrients. Appetite and food choices are generally adversely affected in people suffering acute or chronic stress, which in turn means further nutrient depletion.

ACTIVITY LEVEL

Anyone who exercises frequently to the point of sweating profusely may have an increased requirement for iron and zinc, since these are lost in sweat. Also, since metabolism is enhanced during these active periods, nutrient needs, in general, will be increased.

Exercise is good for the body, but excessive activity depletes the body's stores. Also, intense exercise generates many free radicals, so that the antioxidant vitamins (A, C, and E) and antioxidant minerals (for example, selenium), will be required in greater amounts.

TOXIC LEVELS

The antidiuretic effect of stimulants like tea and coffee means that many nutrients will be easily lost from the body. Smoking and drinking alcohol also increase body requirements for zinc, magnesium, and vitamins B and C because of reduced uptake and increased loss. Any person taking prescribed or recreational drugs, or living and working in a polluted environment, will find their nutritional needs greatly increased because the body requires many nutrients to detoxify these chemicals.

RIGHT Active sportspeople need to replace iron and zinc, as these are lost through sweat.

A HEALTHY BALANCED DIET

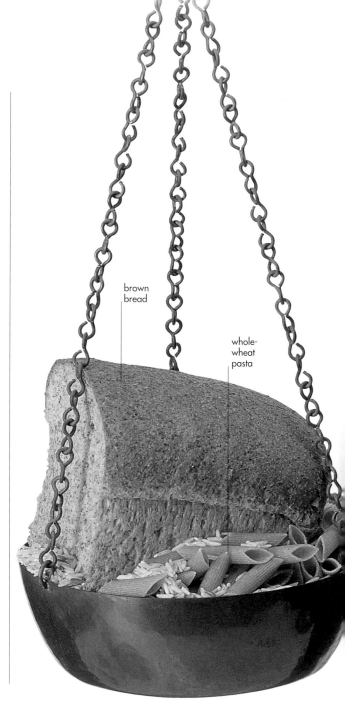

Any healthy diet must include all the nutrients necessary to let the body grow and function effectively, for it to be strong and vital, and for it to resist infection and prevent degeneration. The body must take in sufficient protein for building and repairing body structures. It must ensure an adequate supply of energy (from carbohydrates, fats, and proteins) to maintain basal metabolism and provide fuel for movement. A good supply of water must be available to satisfy the body's requirement for transport, solvent action, fluid balance, elimination of wastes. Adequate fiber is needed for keeping the colon healthy. Vitamins and minerals are required for building and maintaining the skeleton and teeth and for all the hundreds of biochemical reactions that are so important to

LEFT **A good diet in childhood will reap rewards for later life.**

THE MACRONUTRIENTS

There has been little agreement recently about the correct balance of carbohydrates, fats, and proteins—high protein/low carbohydrate/moderate fat; high carbohydrate/low protein/moderate fat; high carbohydrate/low protein/low fat, and so on. At present, the average diet in Britain derives around 44 percent of energy from fat, 15 percent from protein and 41 percent from carbohydrate. In the US, the average diet derives more than 48 percent of energy from fat and roughly 26 percent each from proteins and carbohydrates. Obviously, both of these ratios are unbalanced and not ideal.

The calorific value of the three "macronutrients" differs. Carbohydrates and proteins provide almost the same number of calories (kilocalories)—1 gram of carbohydrate provides 3.75Kcals and 1 gram of protein provides 4.0Kcals. Fat, however, releases almost double these amounts—1 gram will provide 9.3Kcals. This difference means that to balance the three foods from the calorific angle, we should have half as much fat in the diet as either of the other two macronutrients. Also, since we know that high protein diets can be very acid-forming in the body (which can lead to osteoporosis and other disorders), it seems sensible that high protein foods should not make up exactly the same proportion as carbohydrates. However, having a huge amount of carbohydrate (which generally means bread, pasta, rice, and refined carbohydrates) in relation to protein can be just as bad, several recent studies have found that despite us eating high carbohydrate/low-fat diets for a decade or more now, heart disease, diabetes, and obesity are becoming more common.

brown bread

whole-wheat pasta

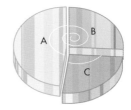

ABOVE The balance of carbohydrates (B), fats (A), and proteins (C) required in the UK.

ABOVE The balance of carbohydrates (B), fats (A), and proteins (C) required in the United States.

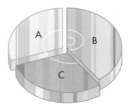

ABOVE The ideal amount of fats (A), proteins (C), and carbohydrates (B) in the diet.

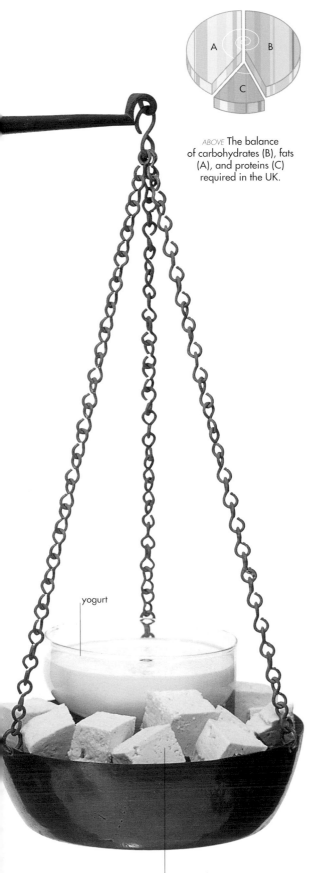

yogurt

bean curd

ABOVE The balance of the diet should be tipped slightly toward unrefined carbohydrates, compared to protein.

The ideal diet, in calorific terms, is one in which a maximum of 30 percent is derived from fat, 30 percent from protein and 40 percent from carbohydrate. If we translate this information into actual amounts of food, we arrive at a ratio of 4:3 carbohydrate to protein (because they supply almost the same amount of energy gram for gram). Since fat supplies double the calories of either protein or carbohydrate, its ratio of 3 is halved to 1.5. The final result is a ratio of 4:3:1.5, or 8:6:3 carbohydrate:protein:fat. This is a much better balance of the three macronutrients than the extremes we have sometimes had in the past.

The types of foods within each of the three groups can have very different effects on your health in general. The best high-carbohydrate foods are those from whole grains and their unrefined products: wholegrain bread, brown rice, and oats. Carbohydrate will also be supplied in the form of starches and sugars from vegetables and fruit. Whole grains and fibrous vegetables, like green beans, will additionally supply dietary fiber. Refined white flour products and sugary processed foods are going to do nothing for your health in the long term.

The best proteins are fish, live yogurt, bean curd, pulses, seeds, nuts, and lean meat and poultry. Fatty meats and products made from these, and high fat cheeses, cream, butter, and even milk, should be kept low in the diet.

The best fats come from seeds, nuts, and their oils (including olive oil), and from avocado and fish. These foods will provide you with the essential fatty acids needed for proper brain and nerve function, a healthy cardiovascular system, good immune function, and good hormonal health. They are also good for joints and bones, and for keeping them working properly: elderly people would do well to increase their intake. Olive oil (or a little good quality butter) should be the only oil you cook with since these are fairly stable when heating; other seed oils should always be used unheated with salads and other foods. Any other source of processed oils or margarines should be minimal in the diet. Most of these heated oils are difficult for the metabolism to process and have many carcinogenic properties.

tomato

yellow bell pepper

red onion

BELOW **Fresh vegetables grown in your own garden, without the use of artificial sprays and pesticides, are the best to eat. Organic food is preferable.**

THE MICRONUTRIENTS

Vitamins and minerals are found in every single item of food we consume, apart from non-foods like white sugar. By far the best way to ensure that micronutrient-dense foods make up the larger part of your diet is to eat a wide range of fresh vegetables and fruit daily, in addition to the correct balance of macronutrients. Furthermore, choosing vegetables and fruit from the color range of red, purple, green, oranges and yellow will ensure not only a good range of vitamins and minerals but will also provide phytochemicals. Many of these have been found to have anticancer, antioxidants and hormone-enhancing properties. Macronutrients will also supply many vitamins and minerals.

THE QUALITY OF FOOD

It is healthiest to choose fresh, organic food. A good-quality soil will contain most of the necessary minerals and trace elements. If it is farmed organically, it will be treated with compost and manure rather than chemical fertilizers or pesticides. Organic livestock eat uncontaminated, natural foods and are not treated with drugs, antibiotics, and growth enhancers. If you live in an area where organic produce is difficult to obtain and you are unable to grow much yourself, then buy the freshest and best quality you can and wash all vegetables and fruits. Adding a little vinegar to the washing water will deactivate many pesticide residues. Remember, even those with no gardens can still grow "sprouted" seeds and pulses on their windowsills.

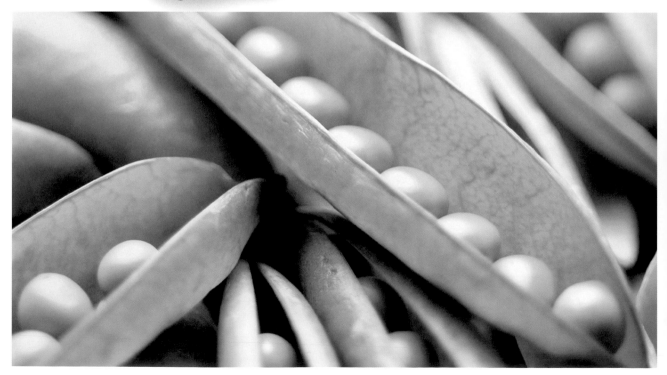

HEALTHY EATING

DAILY

Five servings of vegetables and fruit including at least one from each of the following groups:

- BROCCOLI, CABBAGE, CAULIFLOWER, KALE, BRUSSELS SPROUTS

- CARROTS, PEAS, PUMPKIN, SWEET POTATOES, TOMATOES, WATERCRESS

- LEEK, GARLIC, ONION, CHIVES

- BILBERRIES, BLACKCURRANTS, BLACK GRAPES, CRANBERRIES

- KIWI FRUIT, MANGOES, PAPAYA, PEACHES, PINEAPPLE

WEEKLY

- THREE SERVINGS OF OILY FISH OR, FOR VEGANS AND VEGETARIANS, THREE (EXTRA) SERVINGS OF GROUND FLAXSEEDS OR FLAXSEED OIL

- THREE OR FOUR LARGE GLASSES OF SOY MILK, OR THREE OR FOUR SERVINGS OF BEAN CURD

- THREE OF FOUR SERVINGS OF PLAIN LIVE SOY, SHEEP'S, GOAT'S, OR COW'S YOGURT

- THREE SERVINGS OF MIXED WHOLE NUTS

OTHER VEGETABLES AND FRUITS NOT LISTED ABOVE

- SEA VEGETABLES (EDIBLE SEAWEED) ADDED TO SOUPS, STEWS, AND CASSEROLES

- WHITE FISH

- LEAN MEATS AND POULTRY

- UNHEATED, HIGH-QUALITY SALAD OILS AND DRESSINGS

- ONE OR TWO EGGS

- HONEY, MOLASSES, OR PURE FRUIT JAM

- A LITTLE CHEESE, MILK, AND BUTTER

- NATURAL CONDIMENTS AND HERBS

- A LITTLE RED WINE IF DESIRED

- A FEW TREATS, SUCH AS GOOD QUALITY CHOCOLATE OR A SLICE OF HOME-MADE CAKE

GENERAL TIPS

- For maximum nutrient retention, only lightly cook non-fibrous vegetables and fruit or eat raw.
- Steam or stir-fry fibrous foods such as runner beans and carrots.
- Save cooking water from vegetables to use in soups and stews.
- If frying is necessary, use olive oil, or "steam-fry" with vegetable extract, vegetable or fish bouillon, or miso.
- Keep processed food, confectionery, refined carbohydrates, dairy food (except yogurt), and alcohol to a minimum.
- Avoid saturated fat, heated polyunsaturated oils, white sugar, and excess salt.
- Store all oils and foods containing essential fatty acids (including seeds and nuts) in a cool, dark cupboard (or fridge) in tightly-sealed jars.
- Choose organic food or select foods close to their natural form.
- Eat up fresh vegetables quickly; each day nutrients will be lost, even if stored in a cool place.

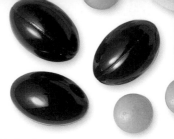

HOW TO TAKE SUPPLEMENTS

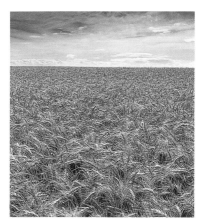

For several reasons it is not always possible to obtain the nutrients needed from food for several reasons. Soil nowadays lacks many minerals because of intensive crop growing and the use of chemical fertilizers. Even organic food, though it obviously has far fewer pesticides and other pollutants, still does not provide nutrients in the amounts which were available in fresh food several decades ago—it will be some time before soil minerals reach healthy levels again.

LEFT Wheat is ground into flour for bread and pasta.

Many people have digestive systems that are not sufficiently effective in breaking down food and absorbing nutrients—they may have poor levels of stomach acid, insufficient production of digestive enzymes, or toxic substances in the gut, among other reasons. (These conditions should improve dramatically, however, as nutrient intake increases.)

Thus, although an organic diet is the healthiest one that we can follow, we may need to compensate for any shortfalls by taking supplements.

Supplements can be self-prescribed and taken in small regular amounts as a form of health insurance or to treat minor health problems. Supplements in larger amounts for nutritional support of severe pathological conditions have been found to be therapeutic either on their own or with conventional medical treatments, but these larger doses should always be taken under the supervision of a nutritional therapist or a physician.

LEFT Small doses of supplements may be safely taken on a regular basis.

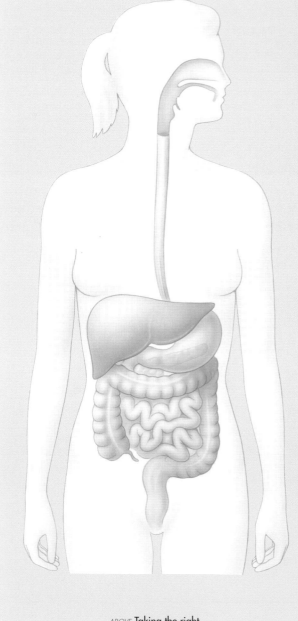

THE DIGESTIVE SYSTEM

ABOVE Taking the right supplements can help your digestive system.

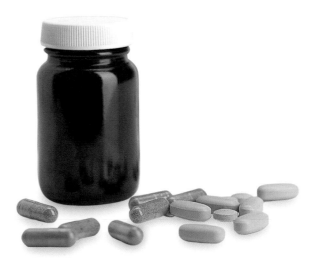

Supplemental vitamins and minerals often contain several times the normal levels, except for toxic ones, including vitamins A and D. Where there is no established safe level, supplements will always contain levels of micronutrients that are very unlikely to cause harm when taken at the manufacturer's dosages. Supplements are available as single nutrients, or are combined sometimes as a broad-spectrum multiformula. So long as you follow the manufacturer's dosage instructions and ensure that you have no condition that is contraindicated for that supplement, then you are likely to have no problems. (Note: Several supplements, usually single substances and herbs, are contraindicated for some conditions, especially for pregnant and nursing mothers. If you have any pre-existing conditions, see your practitioner or physician before taking supplements. Always read the instructions carefully on supplement labels before you take them.) Allergies and intolerances can occur on the rare occasion, but most manufacturers produce hypoallergenic ranges that manage to circumvent this problem.

WHEN TO TAKE SUPPLEMENTS

VITAMINS A, D, E	With meals which include a little oil or fat
VITAMIN B-COMPLEX	First thing in the morning for maximum energy, but safe any time, especially when taken with whole grains
VITAMIN C	With meals, two or three times a day; ascorbate can be taken safely on an empty stomach even in fairly large amounts, as may be appropriate to treat a cold
IRON	Best absorbed with foods that naturally contain iron. But, to prevent interaction with other minerals, it can be taken on an empty stomach; the organic form of iron should not produce nausea
CALCIUM	30 minutes before bedtime
MAGNESIUM	30 minutes before bedtime
ZINC	With a meal; can cause nausea if taken on an empty stomach or with insufficient food
OTHER MINERALS	With meals
MULTIFORMULAS	Any time is effective and safe; can be taken with fluid alone, though would be better absorbed if taken with a small amount of food
TIME-RELEASE	With the main meal of the day.

RIGHT Follow the manufacturer's advice on how to take your vitamin and mineral supplements.

WHEN TO TAKE SUPPLEMENTS

The best time to take supplements is usually with meals; absorption is best when the digestive system has been stimulated by the presence of food. Time-release formulas should always be taken with food to ensure they travel through the body at the correct speed for efficient release at the appropriate place.

The water-soluble vitamins (B-complex and C) pass out of the body fairly quickly, so that small doses taken twice or three times a day are often the best practice. The fat-soluble vitamins will be absorbed better if taken with meals that include some fat. Most minerals work in conjunction with vitamins and should be taken along with them. Some minerals interfere with the absorption of others, so you may need to take them at a different time from your multiformula. If a multiformula contains antagonistic minerals, they will be present in amounts that do not conflict with one another, so you need not worry.

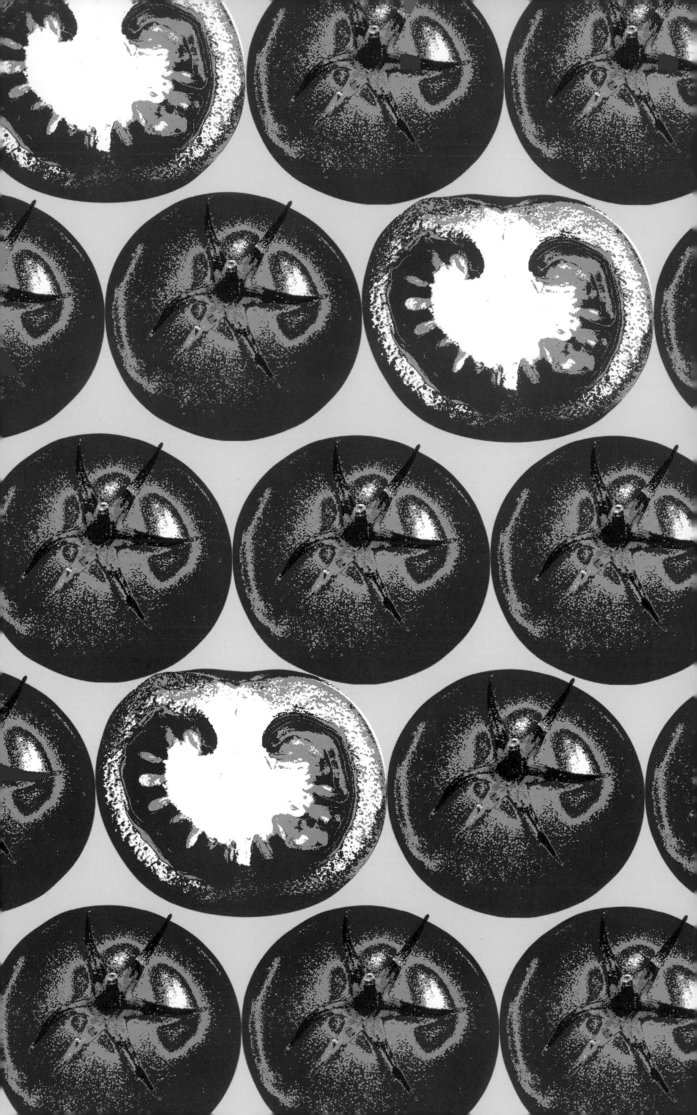

PART TWO

THE VITAMINS

Vitamins are compounds needed by the body in small quantities to help it do its vital work of growing, developing, and functioning. Vitamins work closely with the enzymes in the body, and other compounds, to help produce energy, build new tissue, remove waste material, and to ensure that each system works effectively and efficiently. With a few exceptions—such as vitamin D, which can actually by synthesized by our bodies—the nutrients we need cannot be produced by the body and must be obtained from foods and supplements. In the following pages, the most important vitamins are laid out, along with their function in our bodies, and the recommended dosage of each supplement.

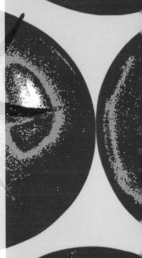
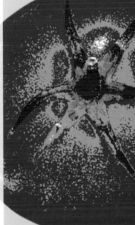
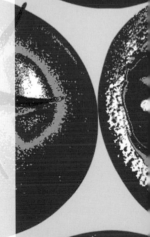

VITAMIN A

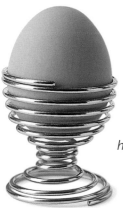

Vitamin A is fat-soluble. Its importance for eyesight originally made it known as the "vision vitamin"; then it became the "anti-infective vitamin" because of its importance in immune status and membrane integrity. Wherever mucous membranes occur in the body—skin, the lining of the nose, throat, lungs, urogenital tract, and gut—they are the first lines of defense against microbial invasion. Vitamin A and its relatives, the carotenes, are also antioxidants, helping to prevent the damaging effects of "free radicals."

LEFT Vitamin A in the form of retinol is found in eggs.

Vitamin A comes in two natural forms: retinol, found in animal products like liver, eggs, butter, and fish liver oils; and beta-carotene, the plant source of vitamin A, found in dark orange vegetables, dark green leafy vegetables, and fruits. Beta-carotene is effectively two units of retinol joined together and is converted to vitamin A by our body (mainly by the liver) when needed.

RETINOL

Retinol gets its name from the retina of the eye. It is the basis of the visual pigment called rhodopsin (visual purple) which needs to be constantly reformed after taking part in the reception of light stimuli. Apart from the use of vitamin A in the diet to treat and prevent various types of blindness, synthetic derivatives of retinol have been developed to treat many skin conditions from severe acne to certain forms of cancer.

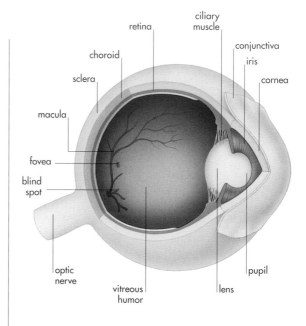

ABOVE Vitamin A, the "vision" vitamin, is essential for healthy eyes.

DIETARY REFERENCE VALUES FOR VITAMIN A			
	retinol equivalents (mcg/day)	rni iu/day	rda iu/day
CHILDREN			
UNDER 1 YEAR	350	1,167	1,875
1–6 YEARS	400	1,333	2,000/2,500
7–10 YEARS	500	1,667	3,500
11–14 YEARS	600	2,000	5,000
ADULTS			
MALES 15 +	700	2,333	5,000
FEMALES 11 +	600	2,000	4,000
PREGNANT FEMALES	700	2,333	4,000
LACTATING FEMALES	950	3,167	4,000

BETA-CAROTENE

Beta-carotene is often referred to as pro-vitamin A. Carotenes represent the most widespread group of naturally occurring pigments in nature. They are fat-soluble compounds of an intensely red and yellow color and are found in all organisms that transform sunlight into chemical energy via the process of photosynthesis. They play a crucial role in protecting plants against free radicals generated during the process of photosynthesis. Both of these functions in plants—a pigment for "trapping" light and a protector against oxidation—indicate the importance of these pigments in our food for eye health and for our protection against free-radical damage.

DIETARY SOURCES OF RETINOL	
vitamin a (retinol) content of selected foods (IU/100g serving)	
HALIBUT LIVER OIL	900,000
LIVER, LAMB	66,333
COD LIVER OIL	60,000
LIVER, BEEF	43,900
LIVER, CALF	22,500
LIVER, CHICKEN	12,100
BUTTER	3,283
CHEDDAR CHEESE	1,210
EGGS	633
KIDNEY, PIG	533
MILK	187
MACKEREL	150
BEEF, MEAT	33
SARDINES, CANNED	23

RIGHT Carotenes are fat-soluble compounds of an intensely red and yellow colour.

DIETARY SOURCES OF BETA-CAROTENE	
beta-carotene content of selected foods (IU/100g)	
KALE	8,900
CARROTS, OLD	6,667
PARSLEY	4,500
SPINACH	3,333
SWEET POTATO	2,233
APRICOTS, DRIED	2,000
WATERCRESS	1,667
BROCCOLI	1,300
MANGO	667
TOMATOES	333
CABBAGE	167
PEAS, FROZEN	167

RIGHT Oily fish is an excellent source of Vitamin A: avoid too much if you are pregnant.

TOXICITY

Vitamin A, as retinol, can become toxic at high levels. It is especially dangerous for pregnant women who should avoid concentrated sources, such as liver and dietary supplements (unless otherwise advised by their doctor). Beta-carotene, however, is an extremely safe form of vitamin A because, at very high intake levels, the body's ability to convert beta-carotene to retinol slows down dramatically. The only known side effect occurring with high levels of beta-carotene is "carotenemia," a harmless condition in which the skin turns a slightly orange color. Reducing the intake of high beta-carotene foods and ceasing to take beta-carotene supplements is the remedy.

VITAMIN A CONTENT OF FOOD

Meat-eaters easily obtain sufficient vitamin A from their diet, particularly if they eat fish or liver on a regular basis. Vegans and vegetarians should have a varied vegetable intake of beta-carotene-rich food. Current research indicates, however, that beta-carotene absorption is much greater if vegetables, especially fibrous ones like carrots, are lightly cooked.

ABSORPTION AND ASSIMILATION

Sometimes, mainly in periods of ill health, it is not possible to absorb maximally from our food. A variety of factors influence the absorptive efficacy of vitamin A and beta-carotene. Unlike retinol, carotenes require bile acids to facilitate absorption. Anyone suffering from conditions that limit the flow of bile may absorb only a fraction of the vitamin A present in their diet. The presence of fat, protein, and antioxidants in the food are all needed for maximum absorption. A normal complement of pancreatic enzymes in the intestinal lumen together with a healthy layer of mucosal (lining) cells is also necessary. The absorptive efficiency of (animal) vitamin A is usually quite high (80–90 percent), with only a slight reduction in efficiency at high doses. In contrast, beta-carotene's absorption is much lower (40–60 percent) and it decreases rapidly with increasing dosage.

The conversion of beta-carotene to vitamin A once inside the body also depends on several factors. These include protein status, thyroid hormones, zinc, and vitamin C. For efficient usage of vitamin A from carotene, other aspects of the diet need to be optimal and a well-functioning endocrine system (hormonal system) is a prerequisite. Therefore, prior work on the digestive and hormonal systems by nutritional healing or other therapy, is desirable to improve absorption of this vitamin, before bombarding the system with concentrated vitamin A foods or supplements in an attempt to heal vitamin A associated symptoms, such as skin and eye conditions. Without this initial work, taking higher and higher levels of vitamin A (either as high vitamin A foods or supplements) may ultimately impair health as other nutrients become unbalanced.

BELOW Oily fish eaten three times a week gives a good boost of vitamin A.

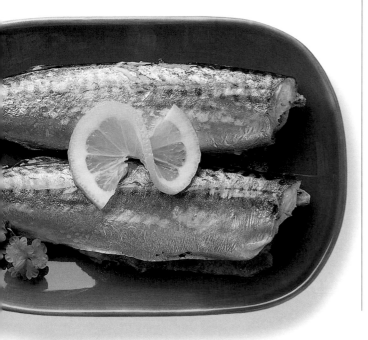

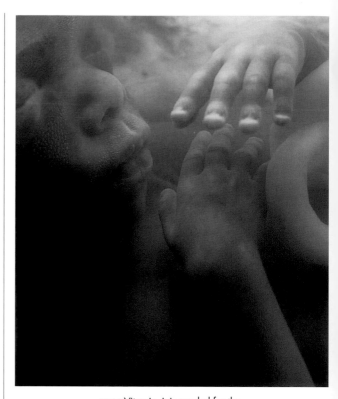

ABOVE Vitamin A is needed for the developing fetus in the womb.

FUNCTIONS OF VITAMIN A

• Maintains healthy skin and mucous membranes—helping to protect against infection of the nose, throat, lungs, urogenital tract, and intestines.

• Enhances antitumor activity, white blood cell function, and antibody response.

• Protects against free-radicals and delays the sign of aging.

• Helps in inflammatory conditions such as arthritis.

• Necessary in the formation of visual purple.

• Needed for proper development of the fetus in the womb.

• Influential in appropriate bone development.

FUNCTIONS OF VITAMIN A

Vitamin A, as retinol or beta-carotene, is required for the growth and normal development of the human embryo and to ensure appropriate differentiation and maturation of all body tissues.

Other nutrients such as vitamin C and zinc are also needed for clear skin and a healthy immune system. Since vitamin A is a nutrient important for a healthy intestinal lining, the common problem of "leaky gut" can often be helped by eating foods containing vitamin A. Indeed, as the gut lining heals with the help of vitamin A, so the absorption rate of vitamin A from foods and supplements is increased.

VITAMIN A SUPPLEMENTATION

For those who are borderline deficient in vitamin A, a substantial increase in uptake will result just by ensuring that the diet is high in the vitamin A-foods or from taking a multiformula supplement that includes moderate levels of both retinol and beta-carotene.

ABOVE Cod liver oil capsules are a convenient way to take in vitamin A.

However, where symptoms are more developed, it may be necessary to take vitamin A (under strict supervision) as a single supplement. Such cases include individuals suffering from: diabetes, hypothyroidism, or severe liver malfunction (beta-carotene is not readily converted into vitamin A in these conditions); fat malabsorption problems; impaired absorption conditions such as celiacs or gastrectomy patients; kidney conditions where excessive amounts of vitamin A can be lost from the body.

CASE STUDY

When a woman's immune system is depressed, she is more susceptible to vaginal candidiasis. Immune depression can be caused by marginal deficiencies in several nutrients, but when symptoms additional to vaginal thrush are present, such as dry eyes, itchy eyelids, "goose bump" skin on the upper arms, mouth ulcers, and dandruff, it becomes more likely that vitamin A is deficient in the diet.

Amanda was suffering from all these symptoms and, in addition, found her energy levels were poor. However, she had no obvious digestive or hormonal problems. Since Amanda was past childbearing age, her practitioner's dietary advice included eating lamb's liver once a week, oily fish three times a week, and at least two helpings of beta-carotene-rich vegetables and fruit a day. She was also given a general multivitamin supplement containing 7,500IU of vitamin A acetate and 8,325IU beta-carotene to be taken once a day. After a period of around four weeks, Amanda began to notice that her energy levels were improving and her skin was certainly less dry and "bumpy." At the end of four months, Amanda's health was much better and her candidiasis had completely gone.

DEFICIENCY SYMPTOMS

A clear deficiency is common in some of the developing countries, particularly among young children, with severe eye problems being the most common symptom. Prolonged deprivation results in death. The most obvious deficiency signs are:

• DRYNESS OF THE CONJUNCTIVA AND THE CORNEA (XEROPHTHALMIA)—CAN LEAD TO PERMANENT EYE DAMAGE.

• SEVERELY IMPAIRED ADAPTATION TO LOW-INTENSITY LIGHT (NIGHT BLINDNESS).

A marginal (subclinical) deficiency of vitamin A will lead to:

• INCREASED SUSCEPTIBILITY TO RESPIRATORY TRACT INFECTIONS.

• MOUTH ULCERS.

• DRY FLAKY SKIN, DANDRUFF, AND OTHER SKIN PROBLEMS.

• A GENERAL REDUCTION IN IMMUNE STATUS; FREQUENT INFECTIONS OF ALL TYPES.

• THRUSH OR CYSTITIS.

• ITCHY EYELIDS.

• IRRITATED INTESTINAL LINING.

• EYESIGHT THAT IS POORER IN BAD LIGHT.

Vitamin A supplements can be taken as capsules, tablets, or in liquid form. Fish liver (or whole body fish) oil capsules will also contain vitamin A. The vitamin will be more easily absorbed if vitamin A supplements are taken along with foods containing some fat. The preparations of most good quality dietary supplements will contain vitamin A as retinol and beta-carotene in the same preparation, but separate products are also available. As a general guide, an optimum range for supplementation is 5,000–10,000IU daily (with a maximum safety level of 25,000IU, supervised by your practitioner). For women during their childbearing years a maximum safety level of retinol is 8,000IU, but again this must be discussed with your physician beforehand. The same caution does not apply to beta-carotene supplements.

ABOVE Carrots are perhaps the most familiar source of carotene.

THE B VITAMINS

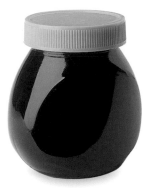

ABOVE Yeast extract is one of the richest sources of vitamin B.

The B vitamins are an interrelated group of water-soluble nutrients that occur together in foods. They are otherwise known as the "B-complex" and comprise B1 (thiamine), B2 (riboflavin), B3 (niacin), B5 (pantothenic acid), B6 (pyridoxine), B12 (cyanocobalamin), biotin, and folic acid. Two other related nutrients, often called "quasi vitamins" since they can be made by the body and are not, therefore, strictly vitamins, are choline and inositol. Jointly, members of the B-complex are responsible for the maintenance of the nervous system, good mental health, energy metabolism, efficient digestion, and many other essential bodily functions.

VITAMIN B1 (THIAMINE)

Thiamine, the first of the B vitamins to be discovered, is a water-soluble nutrient and is, therefore, not stored by the body. It is easily destroyed by overcooking, processing, exposure to air (oxygen), water, caffeine, alcohol, estrogen, and food additives, so it is vitally important to eat fresh, whole foods daily in order to obtain and maintain optimum levels.

Thiamine is essential for energy production, particularly in the brain. In addition to its role as a nutrient, thiamine also demonstrates some pharmacological effects since it is able to mimic an important neurotransmitter, acetylcholine, involved in memory. It has been considered the "morale vitamin" because of its positive effect on mental outlook. As well as its effect on mental functioning, thiamine acts as part of an enzyme called thiamine pyrophosphate, or TPP, which is essential for energy production, carbohydrate metabolism, and nerve cell function.

Thiamine has been well documented as the vitamin that, when severely deficient, causes the disease beriberi. As long ago as the 1890s it was found that feeding fowl a diet of polished white rice produced the symptoms of beriberi, but that by adding back the "polishings" to the fowl feed, the symptoms disappeared. Today, it is common practice to enrich white rice with thiamine and other nutrients lost during processing. However, beriberi is still prevalent in many parts of Asia where white rice supplies up to 80 percent of the total calories consumed by the population. The story of beriberi and the discovery of thiamine highlight the value of whole grains over polished white grains.

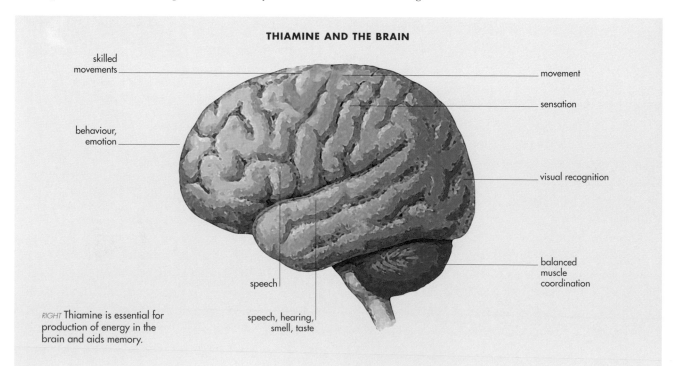

THIAMINE AND THE BRAIN

skilled movements

behaviour, emotion

speech

speech, hearing, smell, taste

movement

sensation

visual recognition

balanced muscle coordination

RIGHT Thiamine is essential for production of energy in the brain and aids memory.

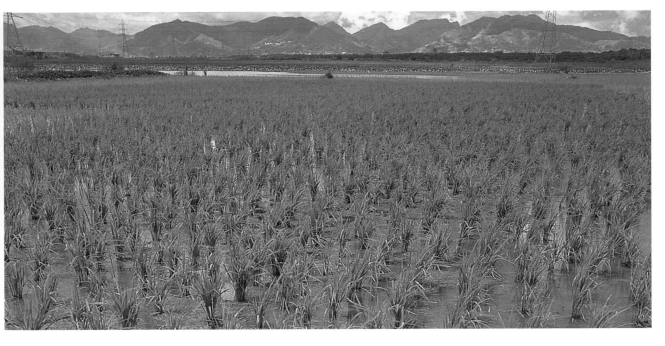

THIAMINE CONTENT IN FOOD

Rich sources of thiamine are wheat germ, soybeans, peanuts, and sunflower seeds; good sources are nuts, whole grains, and pork. Thiamine is easily destroyed, or its absorption in the body reduced, by cooking, food processing, stress, oxygen, alcohol, antacids, tannins and caffeine in coffee and black tea, food additives (especially sulphites), excess sugar, and estrogens. Magnesium, found in whole grains and seeds, is required to convert thiamine to its active form. Anyone who drinks alcohol regularly, smokes, is pregnant or taking the contraceptive pill (or hormone-replacement therapy—HRT), or is suffering from stress needs to increase their intake of thiamine. Also, a cup of tea or coffee with your morning cereals is

ABOVE Thiamine and other nutrients are lost when rice is "polished."

not a good idea if you want to absorb the thiamine present in your whole grains. Eating large quantities of raw fish, blackcurrants, and red cabbage will interfere with thiamine metabolism.

FUNCTIONS OF THIAMINE

It is vital for maintenance of a healthy nervous system (particularly the brain), energy release from carbohydrates, and for protecting against the imbalances caused by excessive alcohol intake. It can help in the treatment of neurological diseases such as Alzheimer's disease and epilepsy. Many patients in psychiatric wards and the elderly are deficient in thiamine.

DIETARY REFERENCE VALUES FOR THIAMINE (VITAMIN B1)		
	rni mg/day	rda mg/day
0–9 MONTHS	0.2	0.3
10–12 MONTHS	0.3	0.4
1–3 YEARS	0.5	0.7
4–6 YEARS	0.7	0.9
7–10 YEARS	0.7	1.0
11–14 YEARS (FEMALES)	0.7	1.1
11–14 YEARS (MALES)	0.9	1.3
15 + YEARS (FEMALES)	0.8	1.1
15–18 YEARS (MALES)	1.1	1.5
19–50 YEARS (MALES)	1.0	1.5
50 + YEARS (MALES)	0.9	1.2
PREGNANCY (3RD TRIMESTER)	0.9	1.5
LACTATION	1.0	1.6

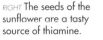

RIGHT The seeds of the sunflower are a tasty source of thiamine.

Thiamine is used therapeutically to help in the treatment of a wide range of muscular and nervous disorders, including lumbago, sciatica, trigeminal neuralgia, facial paralysis, optic neuritis, epilepsy, sensory neuropathy in diabetics, and shingles. It is also frequently used in the relief of postoperative pain.

DIETARY SOURCES OF THIAMINE (B1) MG/100G	
YEAST EXTRACT	3.1
WHEAT GERM	2.0
SUNFLOWER SEEDS	1.9
PEANUTS (WITH SKINS)	1.1
SOYBEANS (DRY)	1.1
BRAZIL NUTS	0.9
BEANS, PINTO AND RED	0.8
MILLET	0.7
BUCKWHEAT	0.6
PORK CHOP	0.6
OATMEAL	0.6
WHOLE WHEAT, GRAIN AND FLOUR	0.5
HAZELNUTS	0.5
BROWN RICE	0.4
RYE	0.4
MUNG BEANS	0.4
PEAS, FROZEN	0.3
WALNUTS	0.3
GARLIC, CLOVES	0.2
PUMPKIN SEEDS	0.2
POTATOES	0.2
CHICKEN	0.1

RIGHT Thiamine can be used therapeutically in the treatment of facial paralysis and neuralgia.

FUNCTIONS OF VITAMIN B1 (THIAMINE)

- Healthy brain activity.
- Energy production.
- Maintenance of nervous system.
- Efficient digestion.
- Carbohydrate metabolism.
- May help in treatment of some neurological diseases.
- Protects against imbalances caused by alcoholism.

THIAMINE SUPPLEMENTATION

The best way to take thiamine is as part of a B-complex supplement. It is available in most nutritional supplements as thiamine hydrochloride. If symptoms are severe, then additional vitamin B1 can be taken at a level of 10-100mg per day, in addition to increasing the levels of whole grains, seeds, soybeans, and peanuts in the diet. There is no known toxicity of this vitamin, though excessively high doses above 100mg/day are not recommended and may cause a variety of symptoms including headache, irritability, insomnia, rapid pulse, weakness, contact dermatitis, and pruritus (itching).

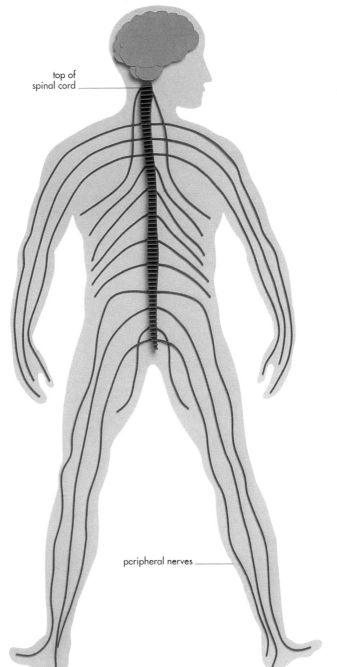

top of
spinal cord

peripheral nerves

ABOVE Thiamine (B1) is vital for
maintenance of a healthy
nervous system.

CASE STUDY

Roger decided it was time to do something about his
constant headaches and indigestion when he began
taking more and more time off work. He had a very
stressful job as a security guard and, to relax in the
evening, he had taken to drinking a couple of pints
of beer with the odd whiskey. Over the last few
weeks, he had noticed other symptoms occurring—
he couldn't get his legs comfortable, his energy level
had nose-dived, and he was beginning to feel mildly
depressed. An article on the B vitamins, and
thiamine in particular, in a nutritional journal
caught his eye; the description of the symptoms
seemed to fit his exactly. Roger began by increasing
the amount of whole grains and soy products in his
diet; he also started to add wheat germ to his
morning porridge and drank fruit juice at breakfast
instead of the usual many cups of tea. His wife
encouraged him to take a B-complex supplement
together with extra thiamine. Several weeks later,
Roger became convinced that his dietary changes
were working, with the help of some additional de-
stressing techniques. As his depression lifted, his
energy level was much improved and even his
digestion seemed better as his daily bouts of stomach
pain and headaches were getting fewer each week.

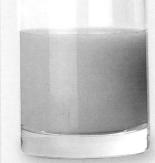

BELOW Add wheatgerm
to a bowl of breakfast
porridge for a
thiamine boost.

DEFICIENCY SYMPTOMS

FATIGUE	PINS AND NEEDLES OR NUMBNESS OF FEET AND LEGS
POOR MEMORY	
LACK OF CONCENTRATION	RAPID HEARTBEAT
DEPRESSION	EYE PAINS
INDIGESTION, NAUSEA, AND/OR CONSTIPATION	MUSCLE WEAKNESS
	LOSS OF APPETITE

VITAMIN B2 (RIBOFLAVIN)

Riboflavin, or vitamin B2, was first recognized as a light-sensitive, yellow-green pigment in milk in 1879. It is a water-soluble nutrient and so is not stored by the body in any significant amount; deficiency is common. It is far more stable than thiamine, being relatively unaffected by cooking processes. Meat and dairy products are the main sources of riboflavin and, therefore, vegans are at the greatest risk of deficiency.

ABOVE **Lamb's liver is a good source of vitamin B2.**

LEFT **Cheddar cheese is a reasonable source of B2.**

The main functions of riboflavin (vitamin B2) are related to its intimate role as the essential coenzymes FAD (flavin adenine dinucleotide) and FMN (flavin mononucleotide) involved in the metabolism of proteins, fats, and carbohydrates, converting them into energy.

Riboflavin plays an essential role in all the oxidative processes on which life depends. A reduced activity of B2-dependent enzymes therefore tends to manifest itself in a generally lowered metabolism rather than in a single or specific block in metabolic pathways. Emotional stress and intensive exercise increase our need for riboflavin, since it is a strong cellular protector against free-radical damage. It is involved in the regeneration of glutathione, a principal antioxidant.

DIETARY REFERENCE VALUES FOR RIBOFLAVIN (B2)		
	rni mg/day	rda mg/day
0–12 MONTHS	0.4	0.4–0.5
1–3 YEARS	0.6	0.8
4–6 YEARS	0.8	1.1
7–10 YEARS	1.0	1.2
11 + YEARS (FEMALES)	1.1	1.3
11–14 YEARS (MALES)	1.2	1.5
15 + YEARS (MALES)	1.3	1.8
PREGNANCY (3RD TRIMESTER)	1.4	1.6
LACTATION	1.6	1.8

RIBOFLAVIN CONTENT IN FOOD

Organ meats, such as liver, kidneys and other forms of offal, are the best source of riboflavin for meat-eaters. For vegetarians, some good sources are yeast extract, almonds, soybeans, and dark green leafy vegetables. Riboflavin is damaged by light, but is not destroyed by normal cooking. However, its activity is dramatically reduced by excess zinc, caffeine, and alcohol in the diet and by antibiotics and estrogens. Requirements increase during pregnancy and breastfeeding and while taking the contraceptive pill or HRT. Because of riboflavin's interaction with alkalis (including bicarbonate), these should not be used in cooking; for example, do not use bicarbonate.

Certain drugs, particularly anti-coagulants, particularly interfere with riboflavin metabolism.

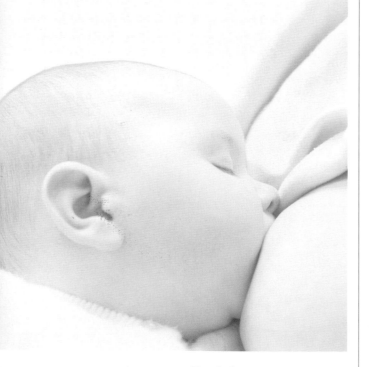

ABOVE **A woman's need for riboflavin increases when she is breastfeeding.**

DIETARY SOURCES OF RIBOFLAVIN (B2) MG/100G	
YEAST EXTRACT	11.0
LAMB'S LIVER	4.6
PIG'S KIDNEY	2.6
FORTIFIED BREAKFAST CEREAL	1.6
ALMONDS	0.9
WHEAT GERM	0.7
CHEESE, CHEDDAR	0.5
EGGS	0.5
MILLET	0.4
SOY FLOUR	0.3
BEEF, STEWING STEAK	0.2
MILK	0.2
KALE	0.2
PARSLEY	0.2
BROCCOLI	0.2
SUNFLOWER SEEDS	0.2
CHICKEN	0.1

DEFICIENCY OF RIBOFLAVIN

Severe deficiency of riboflavin is characterized by extensive cracking of the lips and corner of the mouth; an inflamed tongue; visual disturbances, such as sensitivity to light and loss of visual acuity; cataract formation; burning and itching of eyes, lips, mouth, and tongue; disorders of mucous membranes; anemia; and seborrheic dermatitis. Low dietary levels of riboflavin have been linked to certain esophageal cancers. Riboflavin deficiency is not uncommon in people who have undergone total or partial gastrectomy and those being treated with chloramphenicol, erythromycin, tetracycline, and other antibiotics. Some types of thiazide diuretic can increase the excretion of riboflavin.

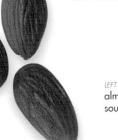

LEFT Whole nuts, such as almonds, are an excellent source of riboflavin.

FUNCTIONS OF RIBOFLAVIN (B2)

• Acts as a coenzyme in converting proteins, fats, and carbohydrates into energy.

• Helps to counteract free-radical damage.

• Aids vision and prevents cataract formation; has been used therapeutically in blepharitis (sore, itchy eyelids), keratitis (inflammation of the corner), and cataracts.

• Maintains the integrity of mucous membranes.

• Promotes skin, hair, and nail health; has been used therapeutically in the treatment of acne rosacea.

• Activates vitamin B6.

• Protects against anemia.

• Helps in the prevention of migraine headaches.

• Has been found effective, on occasion, in the treatment of migraines, muscle cramps, some anemias, and carpal tunnel syndrome.

RIBOFLAVIN SUPPLEMENTATION

Riboflavin is best taken as part of the B-complex at a dose of around 50mg. When symptoms are severe, an additional 10–200mg can be taken. For the prevention of migraine headaches, an amount toward the top of this range is often effective. Riboflavin has not been shown to be toxic at high intake levels; it has poor solubility and intestinal absorption. However, extended use at the higher dosage levels may produce mild numbness and itching and burning sensations. Riboflavin supplementation may cause a harmless intensification of the yellow coloration of the urine.

RIGHT Riboflavin can easily be taken in capsule form.

DEFICIENCY SYMPTOMS	
CRACKED SKIN, ESPECIALLY AROUND THE MOUTH	BLOODSHOT, BURNING, OR GRITTY EYES
SCALY RED SKIN ON THE SIDES OF THE NOSE	CONJUNCTIVITIS
SENSITIVITY TO BRIGHT LIGHTS	SORE TONGUE AND BURNING LIPS
	INSOMNIA

VITAMIN B3 (NIACIN)

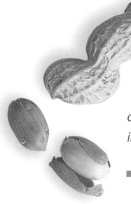

Niacin was discovered during the search for the cause of pellagra, a common disease in Spain and Italy in the 18th century; in Italian, pellagra *means "skin that is rough." We now know that pellagra is caused by a severe deficiency of niacin and tryptophan and is characterized by the "3-Ds"—dermatitis, dementia, and diarrhea—where the skin develops a cracked, scaly dermatitis; the brain does not function properly; and diarrhea results from an impaired mucous lining of the gastrointestinal tract.*

The name "niacin" is a generic descriptor including nicotinic acid and nicotinamide (niacinamide). Both are commonly known as vitamin B3. However, because the body converts the amino acid tryptophan to B3, many nutritionists do not consider niacin an essential nutrient as long as tryptophan intake is adequate.

ABOVE **Raw, freshly shelled peanuts are rich in niacin.**

Niacin is essential in the production of energy, since it forms part of the coenzymes NAD (nicotine adenine dinucleotide) and NADP (nicotine adenine dinucleotide phosphate), which are involved in well over 50 different chemical reactions in the body. Niacin-containing enzymes play an important central role in carbohydrate metabolism and in the manufacture of many body compounds, including the sex and adrenal hormones. Niacin is also involved in the regulation of blood sugar, antioxidant mechanisms, and detoxification reactions. In addition, niacin supplementation exerts a favorable effect on high cholesterol levels.

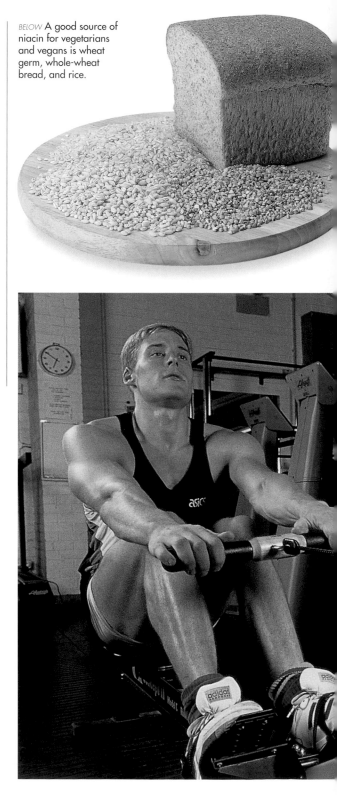

BELOW **A good source of niacin for vegetarians and vegans is wheat germ, whole-wheat bread, and rice.**

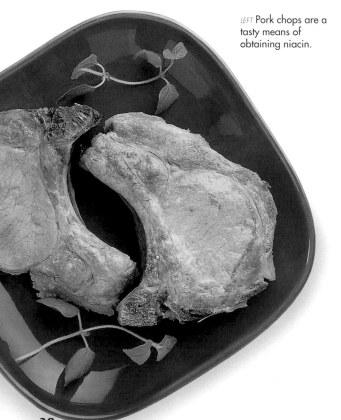

LEFT **Pork chops are a tasty means of obtaining niacin.**

NIACIN CONTENT IN FOOD

Niacin is one of the most stable of the B vitamins, being unaffected by light, air (oxygen), or alkalis. The only appreciable loss of niacin occurs when it leaches into cooking water. Meat and fish eaters should have no problem obtaining sufficient niacin from their diet, and even vegans are able to ensure an adequate level if raw peanuts, brown rice, and seeds are eaten on a regular basis. Niacin may also be made in the body from tryptophan (which is found in bananas). However, this conversion is very inefficient, with around 60 molecules of tryptophan needed to make one molecule of niacin. An exception occurs in pregnant women, where the conversion is twice as efficient. For maximum conversion to occur, thiamine, pyridoxine, and biotin—all members of the B-complex—are needed.

Alcohol inhibits the metabolism of niacin, and sleeping pills, estrogen, and excessive food processing will destroy the efficacy of the vitamin.

RIGHT Most meat and fish eaters should be able to obtain sufficient niacin from their diet.

BELOW Niacin is essential for energy production within the body, as well as being involved in many other essential chemical reactions.

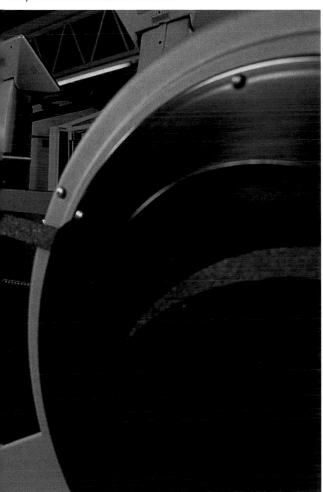

DIETARY SOURCES OF NIACIN (B3) MG/100G	
PEANUTS, RAW WITH SKINS	17.2
CHICKEN	9.6
EGGS	8.5
STEWING STEAK	8.5
PORK CHOP	7.2
WILD RICE	6.2
CHEESE, CHEDDAR	6.2
FISH, WHITE	6.0
MUNG BEANS, DRY	5.5
SESAME SEEDS, SUNFLOWER SEEDS	5.4
BROWN RICE	4.7
BUCKWHEAT, WHOLE-GRAIN	4.4
WHEAT GERM	4.2
AVOCADOS	4.0
BARLEY	3.7
ALMONDS	3.5
FIELD PEAS	3.0
PEAS, FROZEN	2.6
BREAD, WHOLEMEAL	1.8
POTATOES	1.5

NIACIN SUPPLEMENTATION

Niacin is available in nutritional supplements as either niacin (nicotinic acid or nicotinate) or as niacinamide (nicotinamide). It is essentially nontoxic, although doses above 100mg can cause side effects, including the "niacin flush" (caused only by the nicotinic acid form) which is characterized by burning, itching skin and may be exacerbated by antibiotics. If niacin is to be used therapeutically at doses in excess of 100mg, then this needs to be supervised by a physician or practitioner. Extremely high doses of nicotinic acid (3–6g per day), particularly the time-released varieties, may sometimes (rarely) cause liver impairment; niacinamide is considered to be the safer form of niacin, though this is not a useful supplement for all treatments.

For self-treatment, as with all the B group of vitamins, niacin is best taken as part of the B-complex. A level somewhere between 20 and 100mg would be adequate. Single nicotinic acid supplements are contraindicated for people suffering from gout, diabetes, stomach ulcers, and liver disease.

FUNCTIONS OF NIACIN (B3)

Nicotinic acid is concerned with the blood circulation, maintenance of the nervous system, and the reduction of cholesterol and fats, whereas nicotinamide assists in the breakdown of carbohydrates, fats, and protein and is involved in energy production. Both types of B3 are often found together in foods.

• Maintains a healthy nervous system.

• Acts as a vasodilator for efficient blood flow; helpful for treatment of migraines, tinnitus, circulatory disorders such as high blood pressure, and menstrual pain.

• Essential for the metabolism of carbohydrates, protein, and fats to release energy.

• Necessary for synthesis of sex hormones, cortisone, thyroxin, and insulin.

• Helpful in lowering of levels of cholesterol and blood fats (nicotinic acid only).

• Helpful in the treatment of osteoarthritis and rheumatoid arthritis (niacinamide only).

• Helpful in the treatment of schizophrenia and depression.

• Has antioxidant and detoxificant properties.

• Helps in the regulation of blood-sugar.

• Needed for integrity of the skin.

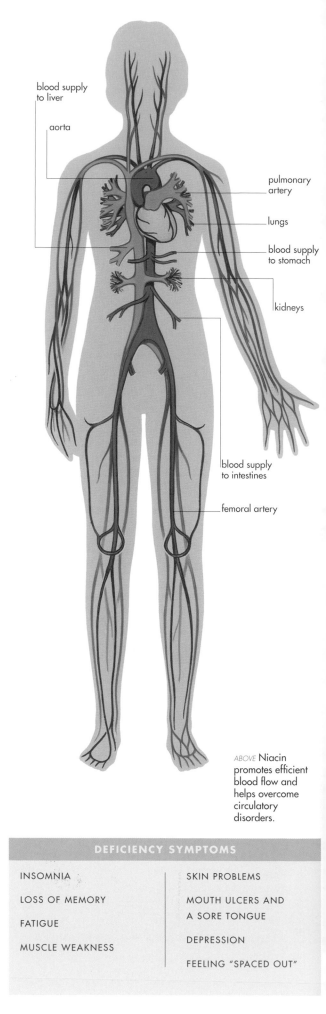

blood supply to liver

aorta

pulmonary artery

lungs

blood supply to stomach

kidneys

blood supply to intestines

femoral artery

ABOVE Niacin promotes efficient blood flow and helps overcome circulatory disorders.

DEFICIENCY SYMPTOMS	
INSOMNIA	SKIN PROBLEMS
LOSS OF MEMORY	MOUTH ULCERS AND A SORE TONGUE
FATIGUE	DEPRESSION
MUSCLE WEAKNESS	FEELING "SPACED OUT"

DIETARY REFERENCE VALUES FOR VITAMIN B3 (NIACIN EQUIVALENT)		
	rni mg/day	rda mg/day
0–6 MONTHS	3	5
7–9 MONTHS	4	6
10–12 MONTHS	5	6
1–3 YEARS	8	9
4–6 YEARS	11	12
7–10 YEARS	12	13
11–14 YEARS (FEMALES)	12	15
11–14 YEARS (MALES)	15	17
15–18 YEARS (FEMALES)	14	15
15–18 YEARS (MALES)	18	20
19–50 YEARS (FEMALES)	13	15
19–50 YEARS (MALES)	17	19
50 + YEARS (FEMALES)	12	13
50 + YEARS (MALES)	16	15
PREGNANCY	13	17
LACTATION	15	20

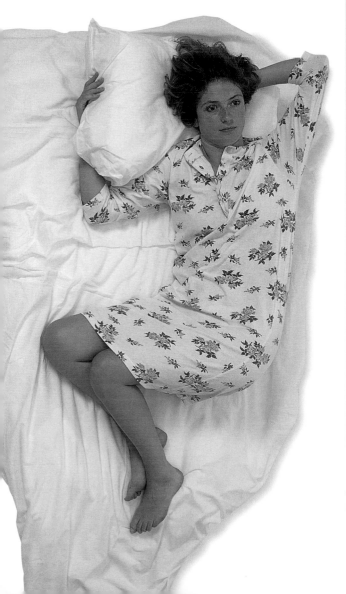

CASE STUDY

Isobel came to see me because she had been diagnosed as having osteoporosis and wanted to optimize her diet to increase her intake of bone-strengthening nutrients. In addition, she was a little concerned about a recent blood test which indicated that her blood cholesterol level of LDL (low density lipoprotein) was higher than normal. Niacin has been found in many scientific studies to lower, specifically, LDL cholesterol and fibrinogen (a blood-clotting substance), while simultaneously stimulating HDL (high density lipoprotein). All of these changes would reduce Isobel's risk of suffering from heart disease later on.

Several changes were made to Isobel's diet, including a reduction in dairy produce to reduce her total intake of fat. She showed concern about her calcium intake. but I assured her that although milk and cheese were very high in calcium, these foods are poorly supplied with other important bone minerals, such as magnesium. Her new diet was to contain good levels of nuts and seeds (especially sesame seeds), which are high in bone minerals, and niacin, to help build strong bones and lower her LDL cholesterol. After several weeks on her therapeutic eating plan, she began to notice some changes in other symptoms that she had suffered from for years but had simply attributed to old age. She had always been unable to get a good night's sleep and one reason for this was that noises in her head (tinnitus) kept her awake, but lately this had become less of a problem and she was most definitely sleeping much better.

Isobel's diet now included whole grains like brown rice and buckwheat, which she had not eaten a great deal of before; since she was not a vegetarian, her weekly menus also included more chicken and eggs. The lessening of her symptoms are almost certainly due to the increased intake of many nutrients, but eating a diet high in minerals and B vitamins is likely to have contributed greatly.

LEFT Older women are prone to osteoporosis. The bones become porous due to a loss of calcium, resulting in brittleness.

VITAMIN B5 (PANTOTHENIC ACID)

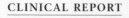

RIGHT **Eggs are a good source of pantothenic acid.**

The name pantothenic comes from the word panthos *meaning "everywhere," since it is widely available in the tissues of all organisms, both plant and animal. It was first isolated from rice husks in 1939. Pantothenic acid has become a popular nutrient over the past decade because of its ability to boost energy levels, improve the immune response, and increase ability to withstand stress.*

Pantothenic acid is a water-soluble vitamin often presented in supplement form as calcium pantothenate. In effect, pantothenic acid and calcium pantothenate are identical. It is one of the safest of all vitamins and, like riboflavin, is helpful in times of stress. The reason for this is its involvement in adrenal function; the adrenal gland is activated by stressful conditions. Pantothenic acid also forms part of coenzyme A (CoA) and acyl carrier protein (ACP). These molecules play a vital role in releasing energy from fats, proteins, and carbohydrates, and in red cell and antibody formation. There is also evidence that this vitamin, in the slightly different form of pantethine, can lower cholesterol and protect against heart disease.

DIETARY REFERENCE VALUES FOR VITAMIN B5 (PANTOTHENIC ACID)

There is no official recommended dietary intake (RNI or RDA) for pantothenic acid, because B5 status is difficult to measure in humans, but there is a "safe and adequate" recommendation

	mg/day
UNDER 6 MONTHS	2
6–12 MONTHS	3
1– 6 YEARS	3–4
7–10 YEARS	4–5
11 + YEARS	4–7

CLINICAL REPORT

Some researchers report that blood pantothenic acid levels are lower in rheumatoid arthritis sufferers. In addition, disease activity appears to be inversely correlated with pantothenic acid levels—the lower the level of pantothenic acid, the more severe the symptoms of rheumatoid arthritis. Correction of low pantothenic acid levels by high levels of supplementation (up to 2g of calcium pantothenate daily) in one double-blind study demonstrated a significant reduction in patients' duration of morning stiffness, degree of disability, and severity of pain. Pantothenic acid has also been considered the "antistress" vitamin because of its central role in adrenal function and cellular metabolism. Its supplementation has produced anecdotal evidence that it helps to reduce stress and clinical trials are in the pipeline.

RIGHT **The adrenal gland responds well to extra vitamin B5 in times of stress.**

PANTOTHENIC ACID CONTENT IN FOOD

Pantothenic acid is found in highest concentrations in liver and other organ meats, eggs, and yeast extracts. Good plant sources include whole grains, nuts, seeds, pulses, and Brassicas (including broccoli and cauliflower). Pantothenic acid is quite delicate and is destroyed by heat, forms of acid (and therefore vinegar), or alkali (and therefore bicarbonate), and is lost through leaching into cooking water. Canning, food processing, caffeine, sulfur drugs, sleeping pills, estrogen, and alcohol all reduce the B5 content of food.

RIGHT Avocados not only taste delicious but also contain pantothenic acid.

DIETARY SOURCES OF PANTOTHENIC ACID (B5) MG/100G	
BREWER'S YEAST	9.5
PIG LIVER	6.5
YEAST EXTRACT	3.8
PEANUTS	2.8
NUTS (IN GENERAL)	2.7
WHEAT GERM	2.2
SOYBEAN FLOUR	2.0
SPLIT PEAS	2.0
EGGS	1.8
OATMEAL, DRY	1.5
BUCKWHEAT FLOUR	1.4
SUNFLOWER SEEDS	1.4
LENTILS	1.4
RYE FLOUR	1.3
POULTRY	1.2
BROCCOLI	1.2
BROWN RICE	1.1
AVOCADOS	1.1
BLACKEYE PEAS, DRY	1.0
CAULIFLOWER AND KALE	1.0

PANTOTHENIC ACID SUPPLEMENTATION

In supplemental use, this vitamin is found as calcium pantothenate. Up to 500mg daily can be used for immune problems and arthritis (taken with an equal amount of vitamin C). Pantothenic acid is normally found in the B-complex formulas in amounts between 10mg and 100mg, but there is no harm in taking it singly for a specific reason—for example, to help with stress tolerance and anxiety caused by stress. There are no toxic reactions known to occur with the taking of pantothenic acid, and no known adverse interactions with any drug. Pantothenic acid can also be applied topically. Good results have been claimed for such applications in the healing of bed sores and varicose ulcers.

FUNCTIONS OF PANTOTHENIC ACID

- Releases energy from carbohydrates, fats, and proteins.
- Involved in adrenal function; helps the body to withstand stress.
- Involved in the manufacture of antibodies and red cells.
- Encourages healing of wounds.
- Prevents fatigue.
- Lowers cholesterol and protects against heart disease (as pantethine).
- Used therapeutically in the treatment of allergic stress reactions, trauma, rheumatoid arthritis, and some anemias and immune problems.

DEFICIENCY SYMPTOMS	
DUODENAL ULCERS	POOR COORDINATION
BLOOD AND SKIN DISORDERS	HYPOGLYCEMIA
DEPRESSION	BURNING FEET AND HANDS, AND TENDER HEELS
FATIGUE	TEETH GRINDING
LOSS OF APPETITE	

VITAMIN B6

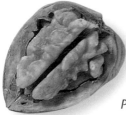

Vitamin B6 incorporates three different substances—pyridoxine, pyridoxal, and pyridoxamine. Of all the B vitamins, B6 is the most important for a healthy immune system to protect against infection and prevent the development of cancer. It is widely used to help relieve the symptoms of PMS and the menopause and has been used in the treatment of infertility. Since it is central to the handling of body proteins, the requirement for it rises with the rise in protein in the diet.

ABOVE **Walnuts are very high in vitamin B6.**

B6 is yet another water-soluble B vitamin that is involved in more than 60 different enzymes in the body. Vitamin B6 helps form proteins and other structural compounds, chemical transmitters in the nervous system, hemoglobin in red blood cells, and prostaglandins. It is critical in its function of maintaining hormonal balance and proper immune function. Vitamin B6 is rapidly converted in the body to the coenzymes pyridoxal phosphate and pyridoxamine phosphate, which play an essential role in protein and fat metabolism. Deficiency of B6 is most common in those of us who eat a diet high in convenience foods, as food processing destroys up to 90 percent of B6 content of food.

Vitamin B6 is necessary for the absorption of vitamin B12; it is often found that the B vitamins work together. This is one of the reasons why they are often found in the same types of food and why, when supplementing, it is important to take B vitamins as part of the whole B-complex.

RIGHT **The symptoms of PMS can be eased by taking B vitamins.**

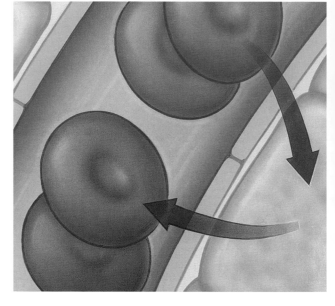

BELOW **Vitamin B6 is important in the formation of hemoglobin in red blood cells.**

DIETARY REFERENCE VALUES FOR VITAMIN B6		
	rni mg/day	rda mg/day
(FOR DIETARY PROTEIN AT 14.7 PERCENT OF ESTIMATED CALORIE INTAKE)		
0–6 MONTHS	0.2	0.3
7–9 MONTHS	0.3	0.6
10–12 MONTHS	0.4	0.6
1–3 YEARS	0.7	1.0
4–6 YEARS	0.9	1.1
7–10 YEARS	1.0	1.4
11–14 YEARS (MALES)	1.2	1.7
11–14 YEARS (FEMALES)	1.0	1.5
15 + (FEMALES)	1.2	1.6
15–18 YEARS (MALES)	1.5	2.0
19 + YEARS (MALES)	1.4	2.0
PREGNANCY	1.2	2.2
LACTATION	1.2	2.1

DIETARY SOURCES OF VITAMIN B6 MG/100G	
SUNFLOWER SEEDS	1.25
WHEAT GERM	0.95
SOYBEANS, DRY	0.81
WALNUTS	0.73
SOYBEAN FLOUR	0.63
LENTILS, DRY	0.60
LIMA BEANS, DRY	0.58
BUCKWHEAT FLOUR	0.58
BLACKEYE PEAS, DRY	0.56
BROWN RICE	0.55
HAZELNUTS	0.54
CHICKPEAS	0.54
BANANAS	0.51
AVOCADOS	0.42
KALE	0.30
RYE FLOUR	0.30
CHICKEN	0.29
FISH, WHITE	0.29
BRUSSELS SPROUTS	0.28
SPINACH	0.28
BEEF, STEWING STEAK	0.27
POTATOES	0.25
PRUNES	0.24
SWEET POTATOES	0.22
BREAD, WHOLEMEAL	0.12
BAKED BEANS	0.12
PEAS, FROZEN	0.10
ORANGES	0.06

VITAMIN B6 CONTENT IN FOOD

Good plant sources of vitamin B6 include seeds, whole grains, pulses, bananas, seeds, nuts, potatoes, and Brassicas. Chicken and white fish supply reasonable amounts for the meat-eaters amongst us. Vitamin B6 is fairly resistant to heat, but may leach out into cooking water. It is also lost by exposure to alkalis or ultraviolet light. Since food processing destroys up to 90 percent of the vitamin B6 content of food, whole fresh foods are the key to optimizing dietary intake.

Any excess dietary B6 is normally excreted from the body within eight hours of ingestion. For this, and other reasons, mild deficiencies are very common. Women taking HRT or the contraceptive pill will have increased requirements, since estrogen destroys B6 activity. Pregnant women are also likely to be mildly deficient in vitamin B6. So too are people with diets high in protein or with an excessive alcohol consumption (the diuretic effect of alcohol will speed up loss from the body). Since some chemicals in cigarette smoke cause diuresis, B6 will be rapidly lost from the tissues of smokers.

The increase in requirement for B6 in the diet appears to have been occurring since the 1950s and seems to parallel the increased levels of vitamin B6 antagonists found in the food supply or used as drugs during the same period. These antagonists include the hydrazine dyes (especially tartrazine), certain drugs (isoniazid, hydralazine, dopamine, and penicillamine), and oral contraceptives. Alcohol and excessive protein can also be viewed as antagonists.

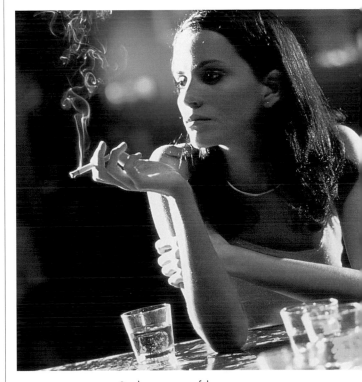

ABOVE Smokers are one of the groups who need to ensure a good intake of B6.

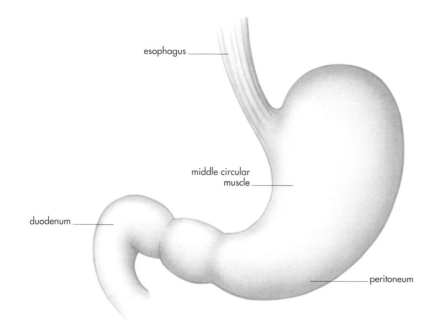

esophagus

middle circular muscle

duodenum

peritoneum

NERVOUS DISORDERS

INFANT CONVULSIONS

SKIN PROBLEMS, RASHES, AND DRY SKIN

SOME TYPES OF ANEMIA

MORNING SICKNESS AND NAUSEA IN PREGNANCY

DIFFICULTY REMEMBERING DREAMS

FLUID RETENTION

OILY SCALING SKIN AROUND SCALP,

EYEBROWS, OR BEHIND EARS

MUSCULAR SPASMS

INSOMNIA

PREMENSTRUAL SYNDROME (PMS)

A NATURAL DIURETIC

FUNCTIONS OF VITAMIN B6

The human body requires vitamin B6 for the proper functioning of many different enzyme systems. It plays a vital role in the multiplication of body cells and is of critical importance to a healthy pregnancy, and in the proper functioning of the immune system, mucous membranes, skin, and red blood cells. These tissues have greater than average needs for vitamin B6 because they are composed of rapidly replicating cells. Lack of vitamin B6 can greatly affect pregnancy and the function of these tissues. Because of its critical role in brain chemistry, in the manufacture of all amino acid neurotransmitters (including serotonin, dopamine, melatonin, epinephrine, and norepinephrine), the intake of vitamin B6 needs to be adequate.

ABOVE B6 is necessary for the production of hydrochloric acid in the stomach.

LEFT A healthy pregnancy depends on an adequate supply of vitamin B6.

FUNCTIONS OF VITAMIN B6

- Involved in the metabolism of protein, carbohydrates, and fats.

- Boosts immunity.

- Balances hormones.

- Helps metabolize and transport selenium.

- Involved in the nervous system (neurotransmitters).

- Helps the body to absorb zinc.

- A natural diuretic.

- Alleviates nausea.

- Promotes synthesis of body proteins and nucleic acids.

- Necessary for the production of hydrochloric acid in the stomach.

- Vital for the production of antibodies and red blood cells.

- Required for the absorption of vitamin B12.

- Useful in the treatment of PMS, the menopause, and in some forms of infertility.

- Protects against cancer.

- Reduces muscle cramps and spasms.

- Prevention of stress-related illnesses.

- Has therapeutic use in morning sickness, insulin resistance, carpal tunnel syndrome, asthma, kidney stones, anemia, fluid retention, childhood autism, heart disease, Chinese restaurant syndrome, depression, immune enhancement, and osteoporosis.

VITAMIN B6 SUPPLEMENTATION

Vitamin B6 is available in supplement form as pyridoxine hydrochloride and as pyridoxal-5-phosphate (P-5-P). Of these, the latter form is known to be the most active. However, intestinal cells remove the phosphate molecule from most of the pyridoxal-5-phosphate ingested before it is absorbed.

Therefore, for most people the pyridoxine form is satisfactory as long as riboflavin and magnesium are also present; these are necessary cofactors for its conversion to P-5-P after absorption. People who suffer from liver disease (particularly cirrhosis), however, may have difficulty in activating pyridoxine to P-5-P, since this step occurs in the liver.

There are various categories of people that tend to be deficient in vitamin B6 and could, therefore, benefit from an increased dietary intake and supplementation. These include:

• Women on the contraceptive pill or hormone replacement therapy (HRT)
• Pregnant women*
• Arthritis sufferers taking penicillamine
• Alcoholics
• Smokers
* Some B6 supplements are contraindicated for pregnant women; read all labels carefully.

Supplemental B6 is also extremely useful in the treatment of PMS, where a dose of around 50–200mg per day seems generally of benefit. The efficacy is increased if the doses are taken in 50mg lots and spaced out over the day. Vitamin B6 has also been used for the prevention and treatment of nausea and vomiting due to radiation therapy, drug therapy, anesthesia, and in sufferers of travel sickness. In all these cases, however, it is always best to take B6 in addition to the full B-complex to prevent imbalances in other B vitamins.

ABOVE Eating a banana is a quick and easy way to get a good dose of B6.

LEFT Alcoholics and smokers will find it difficult to absorb B vitamins properly.

Vitamin B6 is not compatible with the Parkinson's disease medication levadopa, nor with the anti-convulsant medicines phenytoin and phenobarbitone. Doses in excess of 2g daily may cause neurological disorders. Some research indicates that intake doses greater than 500mg can be toxic if taken daily for many months or years.

Owing to recent legislation, supplements are limited to a maximum of 100mg per capsule. If B6 is taken in addition to a B complex, as suggested above, take care that the resulting total dose is not above recommended levels.

CLINICAL REPORT

Low levels of vitamin B6, as well as folic acid and niacin (vitamin B3), have been implicated in the bone-thinning disease of osteoporosis. Low levels of B vitamins may cause an increase in a substance called homocysteine. Increased homocysteine levels in the blood have been found in postmenopausal women (and in some cardiovascular disease patients) and are thought to play a role in osteoporosis by interfering with collagen cross-linking, leading to a defective bone matrix. Further research is required, but so far it has been found that a B6-deficient diet produces osteoporosis in rats, demonstrating that vitamin B6 plays an important role in bone health.

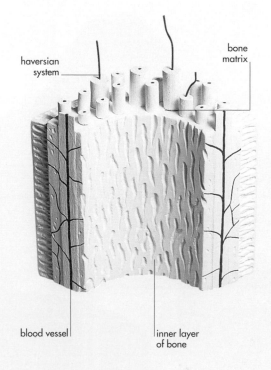

haversian system

bone matrix

blood vessel

inner layer of bone

VITAMIN B12

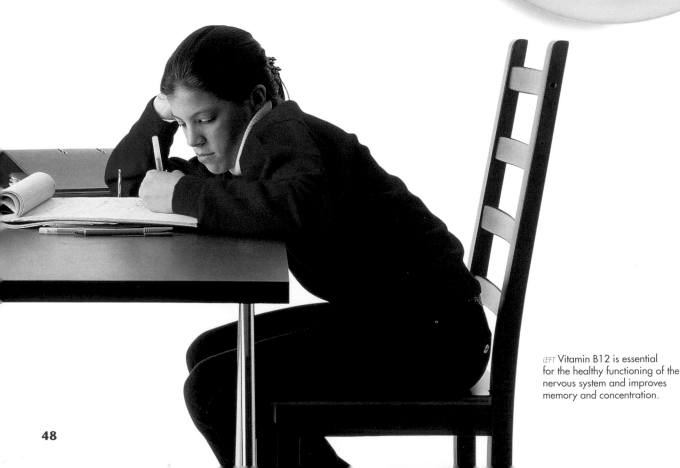

Vitamin B12, also called cobalamin or cyanocobalamin, was isolated from liver in 1948 and identified as the nutritional factor that prevented pernicious anemia—a deadly type of anemia characterized by large, immature red blood cells. Vitamin B12 is a bright red crystalline compound; the color is due to its high content of the mineral cobalt. Like vitamin B1, B12 is known as a "feel good" vitamin because of its intimate role in the healthy functioning of the nervous system.

ABOVE Many breakfast cereals are now fortified with vitamin B12.

Vitamin B12 is a water-soluble nutrient and works with folic acid in many body processes, including the manufacture of DNA, production of red blood cells, and formation of the fatty insulating layer surrounding nerve cells. To ensure good absorption of the vitamin B12 found in food, the stomach secretes a special digestive substance, called "intrinsic factor," that increases the absorption of vitamin B12 in the small intestine. Vitamin B12 also needs calcium to be present for it to be properly assimilated in the body.

Although we need very little vitamin B12, our absorption is often inadequate and vegans, in particular, may need to have fermented foods, fortified foods, or B12 supplements to counteract their low intake.

RIGHT Oysters are a rich natural source of vitamin B12.

LEFT Vitamin B12 is essential for the healthy functioning of the nervous system and improves memory and concentration.

RIGHT Vitamin B12 is fragile and can easily be destroyed, so some people are prone to deficiency. Those who eat fresh fish regularly should have no problem.

VITAMIN B12 CONTENT OF FOOD

Vitamin B12 occurs naturally in animal products, but is extremely rare in plant-derived foods. Shiitake mushrooms are an exception and do contain some. Healthy vegetarians and vegans can, however, obtain reasonable amounts from fermented foods, as many beneficial micro-organisms are able to produce B12. Fermented soybean curd, like miso and tempeh, and fermented milks (including soy milk) are good sources for those eating no animal products. However, there is tremendous variation of B12 content in fermented foods and some evidence indicates that the form of B12 in these foods is not the exact form that suits our body's requirements. Many vegetarian foods are, nowadays, fortified with useable vitamin B12, as are many popular breakfast cereals.

Vitamin B12 is freely soluble and, therefore, lost into cooking water. It is sensitive to strong acid, alkali, and light; alcohol, estrogen, and sleeping pills all act as antagonists toward the vitamin. Individuals who eat fish regularly should have no problem, but there are many people, besides vegans, who may need to supplement their diet in this vitamin. For example, those suffering from intestinal parasites, diarrhea, and other digestive disorders may have very reduced absorption rates of B12. Also, as with vitamin B6, diets rich in protein will need an increased intake of B12.

DIETARY REFERENCE VALUES FOR VITAMIN B12

	rni mcg/day	rda mcg/day
0–6 MONTHS	0.3	0.3
7–12 MONTHS	0.4	0.5
1–3 YEARS	0.5	0.7
4–6 YEARS	0.8	1.0
7–10 YEARS	1.0	1.4
11–14 YEARS	1.2	2.0
15 + YEARS	1.5	2.0
PREGNANCY	1.5	2.2
LACTATION	2.0	2.1

DIETARY SOURCES OF VITAMIN B12 MCG/100G

LIVER, LAMB'S	54.0	LAMB	2.1	FLOUNDER	1.2
PORK LIVER	23.0	EGGS	2.0	CHEESE, CHEDDAR	1.0
OYSTERS	18.0	BEEF, LEAN	1.8	COTTAGE CHEESE	1.0
SARDINES	17.0	CHEESE, EDAM	1.8	MOZZARELLA CHEESE	1.0
TROUT	5.0	FORTIFIED BREAKFAST CEREALS	1.7	HALIBUT	1.0
SALMON	4.0	CHEESE, BRIE	1.6	SWORDFISH	1.0
TUNA	3.0	HADDOCK	1.4	YEAST EXTRACT	0.5

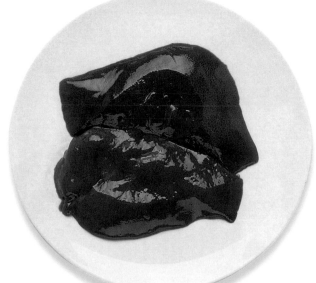

ABOVE Lamb's liver is the best dietary source of vitamin B12.

FUNCTIONS OF VITAMIN B12

Vitamin B12, like folic acid, functions as a "methyl donor." Methyl donors are compounds that carry and donate methyl groups to other molecules, including cell membrane components and neurotransmitters. In this role, vitamin B12 is involved in homocysteine metabolism and prevents its build up in the body. Vitamin B12 also plays a critical role in energy metabolism, immune function, and the workings of the nervous system. It may, additionally, be involved in protecting against cancer and reducing the severity of allergies.

FUNCTIONS OF VITAMIN B12

- Necessary for a healthy nervous system.

- Improves memory and concentration.

- Involved in posture and balance.

- Involved in the production of red blood cells.

- Essential for healthy growth and development.

- Required for the correct utilization of fats, carbohydrates, and proteins.

- Cancer prevention.

- Detoxifies cyanide from foods and tobacco smoke.

- Protects against allergens and toxic elements.

- Useful for alleviating symptoms of PMS and menstrual problems.

- May be used therapeutically for asthma and sulfite sensitivity, depression, diabetic neuropathy, low sperm counts, multiple sclerosis, convalescence, chronic fatigue, confusion and dementia, tinnitus, chronic pain, irritability, and in the treatment of AIDS.

DEFICIENCY SYMPTOMS	
ANEMIA	PINS-AND-NEEDLES SENSATIONS
DIARRHEA	
FATIGUE AND EASY EXHAUSTION	DEMENTIA AND DEPRESSION IN THE ELDERLY
INCREASING UNSTEADINESS, CLUMSINESS,	MENSTRUAL PROBLEMS
	HEART DISEASE
OR TREMBLING	SORE, SMOOTH, BEEFY-RED TONGUE
NERVE DAMAGE	

DEFICIENCY SYMPTOMS

The symptoms of pernicious anemia can be masked if folic acid intake is adequate. This can let vitamin B12 deficiency progress silently, manifesting eventually as irreversible neurological damage. Also, unlike other B vitamins, vitamin B12 is stored in the liver, kidney, and other body tissues resulting in a 5- or 6-year delay (when intake is low) before deficiency symptoms become apparent.

VITAMIN B12 SUPPLEMENTATION

Vitamin B12 is available in several forms, the most common being cyanocobalamin. Supplements of between 50 and 2,000mcg have been reported safe and injections are routinely offered by physicians, especially to those who are lacking "intrinsic factor," though there is some research suggesting that injections are not necessary, and high oral doses have been found to be adequate. Daily

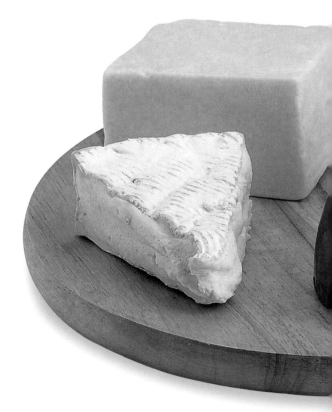

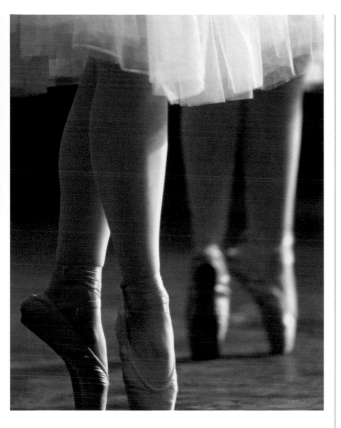

LEFT Good posture and balance are aided by an adequate supply of vitamin B12.

Melatonin secretion also appears to be influenced by vitamin B12, and the low levels of this hormone that are often found in the elderly may be a result of low B12 status. The exact physiology of melatonin is not yet fully understood, but it is known to be critically involved in the synchronization of hormone secretion.

High doses of B12, when administered under strict supervision, have produced good results in the treatment of sleep–wake rhythm disorders, presumably as a result of improving melatonin secretion.

doses are more commonly from 10 to 100mcg, vegetarians requiring the upper dosage levels. Vitamin B12 is absorbed and assimilated better when vitamins A, C, E, and the rest of the B-complex vitamins are also taken as part of the supplemental program. A time-release tablet is often the most useful way to take B12 supplements, since this offers greater opportunity for it to be absorbed in the small intestine.

BELOW Vegetarians who eat cheese will obtain reasonable amounts of vitamin B12.

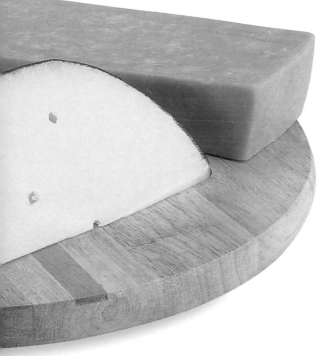

CLINICAL REPORT

Vitamin B12 is vital for correct cellular division and replication, and a deficiency can lead to reduced sperm counts and poor sperm motility. Some research has shown that men with sperm counts of less than 20 million per milliliter, or a motility rate of less than 50 percent, benefitted from high dose treatment of B12 (under supervision), achieving large increases in sperm count, even where observable deficiency of B12 was not apparent.

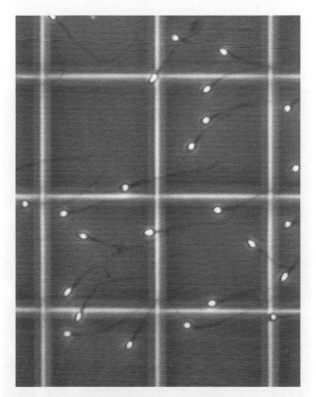

ABOVE A normal human sperm count is about 113 million per milliliter of ejaculate.

FOLIC ACID

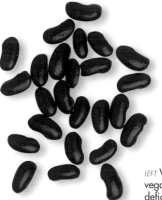

Folic acid was originally found in yeast cells and was recognized as an "anti-anemia" factor. Folic acid received its name from the Latin word folium *which means "foliage," since it is found in high concentrations in green leafy vegetables like kale, spinach, beet greens, and Swiss chard. Despite its wide occurrence, folic acid deficiency is the most common vitamin deficiency in the world. This seems to reflect food choices—animal foods (with the exception of liver) are poor sources of folic acid, while plant sources are rich but not as frequently consumed, at least by meat-eaters.*

LEFT Vegetarians and vegans are unlikely to be deficient in folic acid.

Folic acid is a member of the B-complex, despite it not having been designated a "B" number and is also known as folate, folacin, and pteroylmonoglutamate. It is a water-soluble nutrient critical for cell division because of its role in DNA synthesis and has been identified as being crucial to the development of the fetus. Deficiency of folic acid during pregnancy has been linked to several birth defects, including neural tube defects like spina bifida. To this end, it has been used successfully to prevent infant spina bifida when given at 400mcg or more daily in the pre-conception and early pregnancy periods. Folic acid is also involved in the metabolism of the amino acids methionine and glycine and deficiency has been linked to depression, atherosclerosis, and osteoporosis. It is helpful in the treatment of heart disease and may prevent some types of cancer.

FOLIC ACID CONTENT IN FOOD

Vegans and vegetarians who eat a wide selection of whole grains, pulses, and leafy green vegetables on a regular basis are unlikely to have a problem with low folic acid intake. It is much more a concern for the meat-eaters among us who shun these rich plant sources and plump for eating animal products in preference to these. Babies and young children are at particular risk since they notoriously do not like "greens" and do not commonly eat a wide variety of pulses and whole grains.

Folic acid is easily destroyed by cooking, light, and food processing, so it is often difficult to keep optimum levels as high as they should be. The contraceptive pill, anti-epileptic drugs, antacids, excess alcohol, and aspirin are all antagonistic to folic acid, as too are chemotherapy drugs (especially methotrexate) and sulfasalazine (used in the treatment of Crohn's disease and ulcerative colitis). Oral pancreatic extracts may reduce folic acid absorption, so they should be administered away from folate supplements. Moreover, individuals with an existing zinc or vitamin B12 deficiency are likely to be also deficient in folic acid. Extra folic acid is often necessary when fighting an illness, particularly if this involves the immune system, since this nutrient is used up rapidly when immune cells deal with any type of infection.

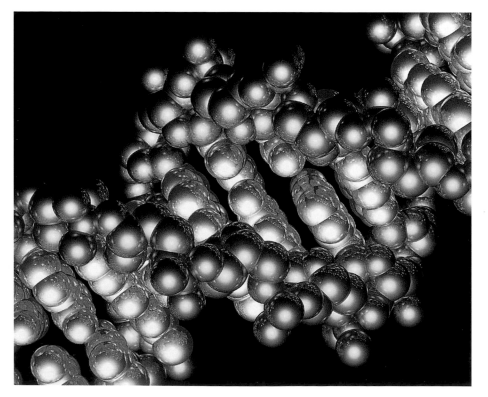

LEFT Its role in DNA synthesis makes folic acid crucial to fetal development.

DIETARY SOURCES OF FOLIC ACID MCG/100G	
BREWER'S YEAST	2,400
BLACK-EYE PEAS	440
RICE GERM	430
SOY FLOUR	425
WHEAT-GERM	310
LIVER, BEEF	295
WHEAT BRAN	260
KIDNEY BEANS	180
MUNG BEANS	145
LIMA BEANS	130
GARBANZO BEANS	125
ASPARAGUS	110
LENTILS	105
SPINACH	77
WALNUTS	77
KALE	70
BEET AND MUSTARD GREENS	60
PEANUT BUTTER	56
BROCCOLI	53
BARLEY	50
BRUSSELS SPROUTS	49
ALMONDS	45
WHOLE-WHEAT, BREAD	39
OATMEAL	33
CABBAGE	32
EGGS	30
AVOCADO	30
GREEN BEANS	28
FISH, OILY	26
DATES	25
BANANAS	22
BLACKBERRIES	14
POTATOES	14

LEFT Asparagus is one of the plant sources rich in folic acid.

DIETARY REFERENCE VALUES FOR FOLIC ACID		
	rni mcg/day	rda mcg/day
0–12 MONTHS	50	25–35
1–3 YEARS	70	50
4–6 YEARS	100	75
7–10 YEARS	150	100
11 + YEARS (MALES AND FEMALES)	200	
MALES		150–200
FEMALES		150–180
PREGNANCY	300	400
LACTATION	260	280

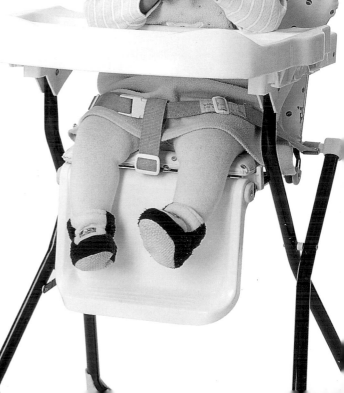

RIGHT It is essential to ensure that a baby's diet contains folic acid.

FUNCTIONS OF FOLIC ACID

Folic acid is needed for many physiological reactions, not least of which is its important role in cell division. All cells of the body are involved, but it is the rapidly dividing cells like red blood cells, immune cells, and cells of the gastrointestinal and genital tract that have the greatest need of folic acid. When this vitamin is low, the results are poor growth, diarrhea, anemia, gingivitis, and abnormal pap smears in women since new cells cannot be produced adequately.

Folic acid and vitamin B12 both function as methyl donors. They carry and donate methyl molecules to facilitate many metabolic reactions, including the manufacture of DNA and brain neurotransmitters. Methyl donation is also involved in the metabolism of homocysteine, a build-up of which may lead to arteriosclerosis and osteoporosis.

DEFICIENCY SYMPTOMS	
GENERALIZED WEAKNESS	REDUCED IMMUNITY
LETHARGY	IMPAIRED MEMORY
IRRITABILITY	NERVE PROBLEMS
EXTREME FATIGUE	SKIN AND GUM PROBLEMS
DEMENTIA	BREATHLESSNESS
NEURAL TUBE DEFECTS	ANOREXIA
RECURRENT MISCARRIAGE	DIGESTIVE PROBLEMS
DIFFICULTY WITH LACTATION	INCREASED RISK OF CANCER
INSOMNIA	

FOLIC ACID SUPPLEMENTATION

Folic acid is available as folic acid (folate) and folinic acid (5-methyl-tetra-hydrofolate). In order to utilize folic acid, the body must first convert it to tetrahydrofolate and then add a methyl group to form folinic acid, so that supplementing with folinic acid bypasses these steps. Folinic acid is the most active form and is more efficient at increasing body stores than folic acid. Despite this, most supplements are in the form of folic acid (folate). The dosage is usually around 400mcg per day, although 800mcg is not uncommon. Up to 5mg is considered safe when supervised by a registered practitioner. Doses of 2mg and over have produced symptoms of skin rashes. Although it is still best to supplement any B vitamin along with all its B-complex relatives, B-complex preparations do not usually contain adequate amounts. In this case, and especially if any of the deficiency symptoms are present, extra folic acid in the form of high-content foods

FUNCTIONS OF FOLIC ACID

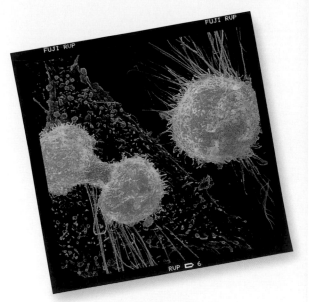

ABOVE All cells in the body need folic acid, specially those that divide rapidly.

• Vital for all cell division.

• Required for the utilization of carbohydrate and amino acids.

• Necessary for red-cell production.

• Necessary for manufacture of nucleic acids.

• Natural analgesic.

• Immune boosting.

• Prevents spina bifida and other birth defects.

• May prevent cancer.

• Improves lactation.

• Essential for healthy skin and mucous membranes.

• Manufacture of neurotransmitters.

• Reduces levels of homocysteine; useful in treating atherosclerosis and osteoporosis.

• May be helpful in treatment of acne, A.I.D.S., anemia, candidiasis, cataract, celiac disease, cervical dysplasia, constipation, Crohn's disease, depression, diarrhea, fatigue, gout, hepatitis, immune problems, infertility, intestinal parasites (including food poisoning bacteria), mouth ulcers, pain, Parkinson's disease, periodontal disease, restless legs syndrome, seborrheic dermatitis, senility, and ulcerative colitis.

CLINICAL REPORT

Cervical dysplasia is an abnormal condition of the cells in the cervix, which is usually regarded as a precancerous state. Some evidence indicates that many abnormal Pap smears reflect folate deficiency rather than true dysplasia especially in women who are taking oral contraceptives, hormone replacement therapy, or who are pregnant, since estrogens antagonize folic acid activity. Some research work on women with cervical dysplasia has indicated that at levels of around 10mg (10,000mcg) per day, under practitioner supervision, folic acid supplementation has resulted in improvement or normalization of Pap smears. Full vitamin B-complex supplementation is also advised.

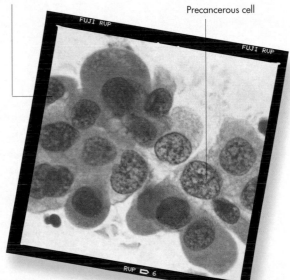

Normal cell

Precancerous cell

ABOVE It has been found that folic acid supplements can normalize an abnormal smear test result over time.

or an additional single supplement may be needed. However, caution must be exercised, since folic acid in excess of 400mcg per day may interfere with zinc absorption, which is another problem.

Much of the benefit of folic acid (plus B6 and B12) supplementation comes from the reduction in body concentrations of homocysteine, which in turn will help to protect against arteriosclerosis and osteoporosis. Supplements of folic acid are highly recommended for the period prior to conception as well as during pregnancy for the prevention of neural tube defects. For the treatment of megaloblastic anemia, folic acid supplementation must be carried out under medical supervision since folic acid can mask vitamin B12 deficiency. In addition to these several reasons for supplementation, other groups of individuals who will benefit from additional folic acid are the elderly, who have poorer diets generally or impaired absorption; those with intestinal malabsorption syndromes; rapidly growing babies and children, where cell division is fastest; anyone on female hormones or drugs as described above; and alcoholics, who generally absorb and retain little folic acid. In cases where vitamin C input is greater than 2g per day or more, extra folic acid will be needed. Vitamin B12 should always be supplemented with folic acid. Vitamin B6 and choline work well with folic acid and may need supplementing at the same time.

RIGHT The wide variety of pulses are among the best sources of folic acid.

BIOTIN

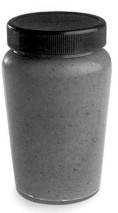

Biotin is a complex organic acid containing sulfur. It was first discovered as part of a complex that promoted the growth of yeast and is found in a fairly wide range of foods. Biotin is manufactured by intestinal bacteria and functions in the human body as an essential cofactor for at least four enzymes. These enzymes are essential in metabolism for transferring carbon dioxide from molecule to molecule, in the breakdown of sugar, fat, and amino acids. They are vital for cell growth and replication.

LEFT Peanut butter is a source of biotin that appeals to most children.

Biotin has also been called vitamin H or coenzyme R. It works together with vitamins B2, B3, and B6 in metabolizing fats, carbohydrates, and proteins in the body and, more specifically, is of central importance in lipogenesis (fat manufacture), gluconeogenesis (glycogen manufacture), and detoxification. It is also the factor that protects against "egg white injury"—caused by eating a large number of raw egg whites which contain a biotin-binding factor called avidin. It is a water soluble nutrient and is regarded as part of the B-complex of vitamins. Without biotin, body metabolism is severely impaired. Since biotin is manufactured in the intestines by gut bacteria, it is usually amply supplied. Also, a vegetarian diet alters the bacterial flora in such a way that it enhances the synthesis and absorption of biotin.

BIOTIN CONTENT IN FOOD

The best sources are organ meats, soybeans, and whole grains. Good sources include cauliflower, egg yolks, mushrooms, nuts, and pulses. Alcohol, food processing, sulfur drugs, and estrogen are all antagonists. Long-term use of antibiotics increases the requirements for biotin, since the body's natural biotin-producing gut flora are

FUNCTIONS OF BIOTIN

- Essential for the metabolism of fats, carbohydrates, and proteins.

- Essential for cell growth and replication.

- Necessary for growth and health of skin, hair, nails, nerves, sex glands, and bone marrow.

- Necessary for energy production.

- Prevents premature graying of hair and baldness.

- Important in the muscle activity.

- Used therapeutically for hair loss, muscle pains, eczema, dermatitis and other skin problems, and some types of diabetes.

destroyed by antibiotics. Biotin works synergistically with other B vitamins, especially B2, B3, and B6, and with vitamin A, as well as with coenzyme Q10 and carnitine (an amino acid). A good vegetarian diet will supply all of these with the exception of carnitine, which is found mainly in meat.

RIGHT Biotin is necessary for healthy hair.

DIETARY REFERENCE VALUES FOR BIOTIN	
Current knowledge allows only for "safe and adequate intake" recommendations	
	mcg/day
UNDER 6 MONTHS	10
6–12 MONTHS	15
1–3 YEARS	20
4–6 YEARS	25
7–10 YEARS	30
11+ YEARS	30–300

DIETARY SOURCES OF BIOTIN MCG/100G					
BREWER'S YEAST	80	LIVER, PIG	27	WHEAT-GERM	12
SOY FLOUR	70	OATMEAL	24	BROWN RICE, WHOLE	12
BROWN RICE (GERM AND BRAN)	60	BLACK-EYE PEAS	21	CHICKEN	10
PEANUT BUTTER	39	ALMONDS	18	LAMB	6
WALNUTS	37	CAULIFLOWER	17	BREAD, WHOLE-WHEAT	6
KIDNEY, PIG	32	MUSHROOMS	16	FISH, OILY	5
BARLEY	31	WHEAT BRAN	14	MILK	2
YEAST EXTRACT	27	LENTILS	13	CHEESE	2
PECANS	27	EGGS, COOKED (EACH)	12		

DEFICIENCY SYMPTOMS

Specific biotin deficiency is rare in adults except those who routinely consume large amounts of raw egg, especially egg whites. The symptoms shown are a type of scaly dermatitis and hair loss. Biotin deficiency is more common in babies, especially where levels of gut flora are low, and leads to skin conditions like seborrhoeic dermatitis (cradle cap) and Leiner's disease.

RIGHT Biotin synthesis and absorption is enhanced by a vegetarian diet.

DEFICIENCY SYMPTOMS	
ECZEMA	POOR FAT METABOLISM
HAIR LOSS	DEPRESSION
PREMATURE GRAYING OF HAIR	NAUSEA
	ANOREXIA
FATIGUE	

BIOTIN SUPPLEMENTATION

Biotin is available commercially either as an isolated biotin or as biocytin—a biotin complex obtained from brewer's yeast. It may prevent the yeast *Candida* from changing to its invasive fungal form and could be useful in the treatment of candidiasis. Biotin has been administered to infants in dosages up to 40mg without side effects and so is regarded as a perfectly safe vitamin even at very high levels. Infants with biotin-deficiency skin problems, who are not breastfed, would be helped further by being given the probiotic *Bifidobacterium bifidum* and fructo-oligosaccharides (FOS) to establish normal gut flora, as well as biotin. Biotin is found in most B-complex supplements and multivitamins at doses ranging from 25 to 500mcg per day. Levels of up to 1,000mcg/day may be used under the supervision of a registered practitioner.

CLINICAL REPORT

Biotin is a popular supplement for increasing the strength of nails and hair. In the 1940s, researchers demonstrated the possible relationship between B-complex vitamins and nail brittleness. More recent work has focused on biotin in this regard. Some data has shown that biotin supplementation at a level of 2,500mcg/day can produce as much as a 25 percent increase in the thickness of the nail plate. The beneficial use of biotin on hair health is possibly related to the ability of this vitamin to improve production of scalp oils—similar to how it works in the treatment of dermatitis.

Biotin supplementation has also been reported to enhance insulin sensitivity and increase the activity of liver enzymes that utilize glucose. The enzyme glucokinase is the enzyme responsible for the first step in this glucose pathway. Concentrations of glucokinase have been found to be very low in those who suffer from diabetes.

CHOLINE AND INOSITOL

Choline and inositol are loosely classified as B-complex factors, but they are not in fact true vitamins because they can be made in the body from other materials and it is for this reason that there are no RNIs or safe and adequate recommendations for choline and inositol. Despite this, choline has recently been designated an essential nutrient and there are supplements available.

ABOVE Citrus fruit contains inositol.

Choline and inositol are both components of various phospholipid structures within cell membranes and are required for the proper metabolism of fats. Without them, fats become trapped in the liver, where they block metabolism. Their lipotropic effect is critical to the health of the liver because stagnation of fat and bile is associated with the development of more serious liver disorders like cirrhosis. Choline is essential in the manufacture of the neurotransmitter acetylcholine—enabling nerve impulse transmission along nerve fibers. Inositol, too, is necessary for proper nerve, brain, and muscle function, since it functions to mediate a cell's response to certain stimuli. It is also found at high concentrations in male reproductive organs and particularly in semen.

Choline is found in foods as lecithin, in the yolks of eggs, and in grains, pulses, and particularly soy. Inositol is present in food mainly as a fibrous material known as phytic acid (inositol phosphate). Phytic acid has excellent anticancer properties and this may be one of the reasons why a high-fiber diet is protective against many of the different types of cancer.

CHOLINE AND INOSITOL CONTENT IN FOOD

Good sources of choline are found in grains, pulses, soy, and egg yolks, primarily as lecithin (phosphatidylcholine) and as free choline in vegetables (especially cauliflower and lettuce), whole grains, and liver. Choline also helps the body conserve carnitine and folic acid. Inositol is present mainly as a fiber (phytic acid) in foods such as citrus fruits, whole grains, nuts, seeds, and pulses. Inositol is liberated from phytic acid by the action of intestinal bacteria.

FUNCTIONS OF CHOLINE AND INOSITOL

• Help in the removal of fat and bile from the liver.
• Vital for the proper transmission of nerve impulses and reception to stimuli.
• Help in the enhancement of memory.
• Form vital structures in all cell membranes.
• Involved in the metabolism of fats and cholesterol.
• Involved in male reproductive organs.
• Used therapeutically in the treatment of liver disorders, alcoholism, arteriosclerosis, memory enhancement, Alzheimer's disease, high cholesterol levels, hair problems, eczema, depression, anxiety, and diabetic neuropathy.

FOOD SOURCES OF CHOLINE AND INOSITOL MG/100G		
	CHOLINE	INOSITOL
LIVER, DESICCATED	2,170	1,100
HEART, BEEF	1,720	1,600
LIVER	650	340
BEEF STEAK	600	260
BREWER'S YEAST	300	50
NUTS	220	180
PULSES	120	160
CITRUS FRUITS	85	210
BREAD, WHOLE-WHEAT	80	100
BANANAS	44	120

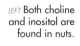

LEFT Both choline and inositol are found in nuts.

CHOLINE AND INOSITOL SUPPLEMENTATION

Choline is available as a soluble salt—in the form of choline bitartrate, citrate, or chloride—or as phosphatidylcholine in lecithin. Most commercial lecithin is low in phosphatidylcholine and may be associated with anorexia, nausea, abdominal bloating, gastrointestinal pain, and diarrhea when very high lecithin doses are given. Newer preparations containing high levels of phosphatidylcholine are now becoming available, which have many fewer side effects.

Inositol is available as inositol monophosphate and is used therapeutically to help liver disorders, depression, panic disorders, and diabetes. No toxic dose has ever been reported with inositol, but high dose choline may make depression worse. Despite some conflicting responses of choline and inositol, at usual dosage of between 50 and 1,000mg (when no side effects occur), they are normally both supplemented together with the other B vitamins. Choline and inositol may be used in supplement form to remove deposited or circulating fats from the body. People with fatty liver or atherosclerotic plaques may particularly benefit. However, these supplements are not designed as slimming aids, no matter how appropriate they may seem.

CLINICAL REPORT

Inositol is required for the proper action of several brain neurotransmitters, including serotonin and acetylcholine. A reduction of levels of inositol in the brain may induce depression. The cerebrospinal fluid of patients suffering from depression has been shown to have low inositol levels. Several pieces of research carried out recently have indicated that in double-blind, placebo-controlled studies, inositol, administered at high doses, has a significant antidepressant effect without demonstrating any side effects. Inositol has also been found to reduce the frequency of panic attacks.

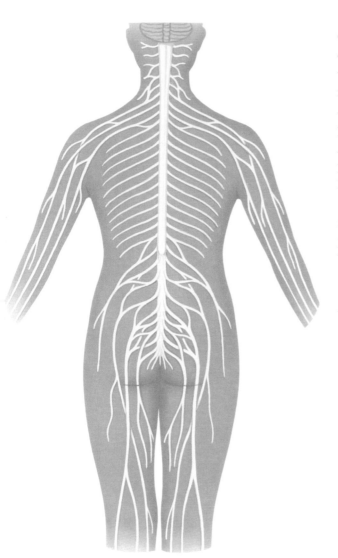

ABOVE Choline and inositol are vital for the transmission of nerve impulses.

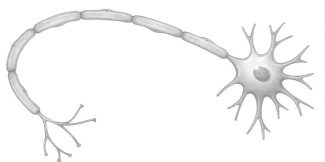

ABOVE The complex network of nerves in the body need choline and inositol to function.

DEFICIENCY SYMPTOMS

CHOLINE	INOSITOL
LIVER-RELATED PROBLEMS	ECZEMA
RETARDED GROWTH	
CIRCULATORY PROBLEMS	
MEMORY IMPAIRMENT	

VITAMIN C

Vitamin C, or ascorbic acid, was first isolated in 1928, though the link between scurvy and vitamin C had been confirmed as long ago as 1768. Today, researchers are still discovering health-promoting benefits for ascorbic acid. It is now the most common nutrient to be supplemented in both the United Kingdom and the United States, despite being one of the most controversial.

LEFT Parsley is one of the best sources of vitamin C.

Humans, apes, and guinea pigs are the only mammals that do not manufacture their own vitamin C and, consequently, remain dependent upon their intake from fresh foods each day. Excess vitamin C is, however, rapidly excreted from the body and easily lost from foods when cooked, prepared, processed, or stored for long periods, especially if exposed to air (for example, after shredding vegetables). A sufficient daily level of vitamin C is derived from at least four or five servings of fresh or lightly cooked vegetables and fresh, raw fruits.

Throughout history, humans have suffered from scurvy, the classic symptoms of which are bleeding gums, poor wound-healing, and extensive bruising. In addition, depression and susceptibility to infection are frequent hallmarks of vitamin C deficiency. Many ancient Egyptians, Greeks, and Romans were affected by scurvy, and this undoubtedly shaped world history as the healthiest fighting forces would be those having access to fresh vegetables and fruit.

Scurvy is rare today, but subclinical vitamin C deficiency is common, especially in the elderly, the young who are institutionalized, and in cancer patients.

Much research has been undertaken on vitamin C, there are opposing views on how much of it we need to consume and the degree to which it should be supplemented in the diet, if at all. Most people think that citrus fruits are the best source of vitamin C, but many vegetables contain higher levels including, broccoli, peppers, parsley, and Brussels sprouts. Many fruits like guavas, blackcurrants, and rose hips also contain more vitamin C than citrus fruits.

Vitamin C is one of the most important vitamins involved in immune physiology and, since it is vital for the integrity of cells, is needed by every tissue in the body. It is, like the B vitamins, water-soluble, and for this reason our bodies are unable to store it; adequate quantities must be provided on a daily basis.

DIETARY REFERENCE VALUES FOR VITAMIN C

	rni mg/day	rda mg/day
0-12 MONTHS	25	30–35
1-10 YEARS	30	40–45
11-14 YEARS	35	50
15 + YEARS	40	60
PREGNANCY	50	70
LACTATION	70	95

VITAMIN C CONTENT IN FOOD

The main sources of vitamin C in the diet are green vegetables, fruits and their juice, tomatoes, and potatoes. However, the ascorbic acid content varies widely depending upon the season, their botanical variety, and the degree of freshness. For example, while potatoes from an October–December crop may contain as much as 19mg/100g, those from a March–May crop may contain only 8mg/100g. In addition, vitamin C is readily lost from foods, particularly if they have been stored for long periods, boiled, processed, or left exposed to air. Its activity is destroyed by oxygen, metals, alkalis, heat, or light. It is important therefore, to eat fresh foods as quickly as possible after their picking and preparation. Although a salad from a salad bar is healthier than a burger and fries, the vitamin C content

LEFT Rose hips have a higher vitamin C content than citrus fruits.

DIETARY SOURCES OF VITAMIN C MG/100G					
GUAVAS	242	PAPAYAS	56	OYSTERS	30
BLACKCURRANTS	200	CABBAGE, GREEN AND WHITE	55	LIMA BEANS, YOUNG	28
PEPPERS, RED BELL	190	SPINACH	51	BLACK-EYE PEAS	29
KALE	186	ORANGES AND JUICE	50	SOYBEANS	29
PARSLEY	172	LEMON JUICE	46	GREEN PEAS	27
PEPPERS, GREEN SWEET	128	GRAPEFRUIT AND JUICE	38	RADISHES	26
BROCCOLI	113	ELDERBERRIES	36	RASPBERRIES	25
BRUSSELS SPROUTS	102	LIVER, CALF	36	YELLOW SUMMER SQUASH	25
MUSTARD GREENS	97	TURNIPS	36	SWEET POTATOES	25
MANGO	80	PEACH	34	LOGANBERRIES	24
WATERCRESS	79	ASPARAGUS	33	TOMATOES	23
CAULIFLOWER	78	CANTALOUPE	33	POTATOES, NEW	16
CABBAGE, RED	61	GREEN ONIONS	32	LETTUCE	15
STRAWBERRIES	59	TANGERINES	31	BANANAS	10

ABOVE Raspberries have a high vitamin C content—almost as much as an orange!

of the salad vegetables in a salad bar will be only a fraction of what it would be in a fresh salad. Freshly sliced cucumber will lose around 45 percent of its vitamin C if left standing for two or three hours. In fact, vegetables like peas which are picked and rapidly frozen will retain more of their vitamin C (so long as they are defrosted and cooked quickly) than fresh produce which has been stored at the greengrocers or supermarket for a while.

Anyone who takes the contraceptive pill or aspirin, who smokes, is stressed, suffers from infections, or who drinks alcohol regularly will have an increased need for vitamin C. Smokers or those who drink heavily, and especially if they do both of these, should have at least an extra 400mg per day above normal requirements. Since carbon monoxide, from car exhaust fumes, is able to destroy vitamin C rapidly, anyone living or working in polluted areas will have increased requirements. Concentrated physical activity, especially if carried out regularly, means vitamin C will be needed to counteract free radicals (produced more rapidly when physical activity is extreme) and to replenish the tissues with this nutrient. Joggers and runners who regularly run along main roads and are exposed to car fumes and pollution will have double the need.

Vitamin C is intricately involved with other nutrients, especially those that act as antioxidants—vitamin E, selenium, and beta-carotene. Also, it increases the absorption of iron, decreases the absorption of copper, and interferes with the blood test for vitamin B12. It is always a good idea to drink citrus fruit juice with your morning egg to aid the uptake of iron from the egg, rather than to have your egg with coffee or tea, which will result in much less iron being absorbed.

RIGHT Limes were given to sailors to combat scurvy on long voyages in the eighteenth century.

FUNCTIONS OF VITAMIN C

Essential and undisputed roles of vitamin C include the prevention of scurvy and helping wounds to heal. It also assists in the absorption of iron and, because of its potential for dealing with destructive free radicals, it is an important antioxidant. Conversely, vitamin C may exhibit pro-oxidant properties in the presence of certain metals and oxygen. These combined antioxidant and pro-oxidant activities are reflected in its function as a co-factor, mediator, or protector in many enzymatic reactions. Consequently, vitamin C has many and varied functions in the body, some of which are still not completely understood.

One major function is the manufacture of collagen, the main ingredient of all connective tissue— ligament, tendon, bone, and skin. This important protein holds the body together and is, therefore, vital for wound repair, healthy gums, and the protection of blood vessels to prevent easy bruising. Additionally, vitamin C is critical to proper immune function and the manufacture of important substances for the nervous system and hormonal system to function correctly.

VITAMIN C AND THE IMMUNE SYSTEM

Many claims have been made about the role of vitamin C in enhancing the immune system, particularly with regard to the prevention and treatment of the common cold and other flu-type illnesses. However, there appears to be conflicting evidence for this, and some research has indicated that the ingestion of vitamin C can actually have a negative effect on the common cold.

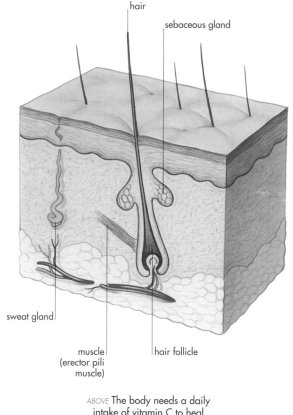

hair

sebaceous gland

sweat gland

muscle
(erector pili
muscle)

hair follicle

ABOVE The body needs a daily intake of vitamin C to heal wounds and repair tissues.

Critics argue, though, that these studies use it at too low a level for it to actually be effective. From a biochemical viewpoint, there is considerable evidence that vitamin C plays a vital role in many immune mechanisms. Normal high concentrations are found in the white blood cells, particularly those known as lymphocytes; infection rapidly depletes this and a deficiency may occur if the levels are not replenished quickly. Vitamin C also works to increase the levels of a substance called interferon, which is made by the cells when under viral attack. Vitamin C is intimately involved in antibody responses, antibody levels, secretion of hormones from the thymus gland, and natural anticancer activity. During times of stress—emotional, psychological, physiological, or chemical—the urinary system excretes vitamin C at a very high rate, making its intake even more crucial. Cigarette smoke, pollutants, and allergens are all examples of substances which cause chemical stress to the body and increased vitamin C intake is recommended. In certain cases, supplementing the diet with vitamin C

LEFT Fruit juices are among the most delicious sources of vitamin C, and can be drunk on a daily basis.

CONDITIONS THAT CAN BE HELPED WITH VITAMIN C

ASTHMA	CORONARY ARTERY DISEASE	HEMORRHAGIC DISORDERS	OSTEOARTHRITIS
ALLERGIES			PARKINSON'S DISEASE
ANEMIA	DIABETES	HEPATITIS	PERIODONTAL DISEASE
ATHEROSCLEROSIS	DUODENAL ULCERS	HERPES INFECTIONS	PEPTIC ULCERS
AUTO-IMMUNE DISORDERS	ECZEMA	HIGH BLOOD PRESSURE	PRE-ECLAMPSIA OF PREGNANCY
	ELEVATED CHOLESTEROL LEVELS	INFERTILITY	
CANCER THERAPY		LOW SPERM COUNTS	RHEUMATOID ARTHRITIS
CANDIDIASIS	FATIGUE	MANIC DEPRESSION	SKIN ULCERS, BURNS, AND WOUND- HEALING PROBLEMS
CATARACTS	FRACTURES	MACULAR DEGENERATION	
CERVICAL DYSPLASIA	GALL BLADDER DISEASE	MENOPAUSE PROBLEMS	SPORTS INJURIES
COMMON COLD	GINGIVITIS	MITRAL VALVE PROLAPSE	SURGERY
CROHN'S DISEASE	GLAUCOMA	MULTIPLE SCLEROSIS	TOXICITY

is the only way to increase the levels to a high enough state to counteract the processes that deplete the body of this important nutrient.

THERAPEUTIC USES OF VITAMIN C

Numerous experimental studies indicate that vitamin C benefits the body in a plethora of ways. It has been used in cancer prevention—especially of the stomach, esophagus, mouth, breast, cervix, pancreas, and colon.

FUNCTIONS OF VITAMIN C

- Formation of antibodies.

- Stimulation of white blood cells.

- Formation of collagen.

- Tissue repair and wound-healing.

- Formation of corticosteroid hormones in the adrenal glands (stress hormones).

- Oxidation of certain amino acids, including tyrosine and carnitine.

- Absorption and assimilation of iron.

- Metabolism of folic acid.

- Antioxidant activity.

- Maintains healthy blood vessels, skin, gums, bones, and teeth.

- Acts as a natural antihistamine.

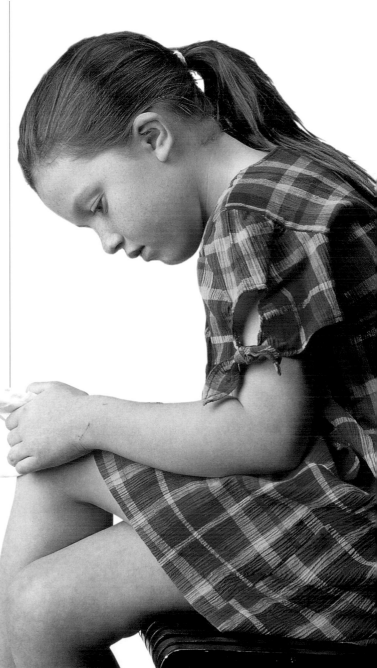

RIGHT Vitamin C is essential to maintain healthy hair and skin.

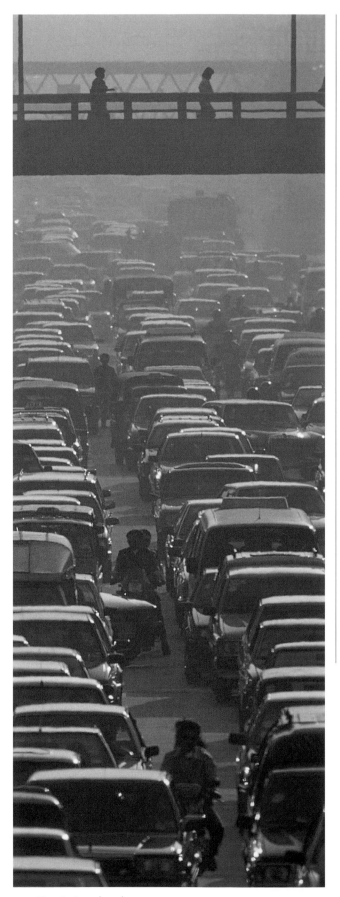

ABOVE Vitamin C combats the chemical stress caused by traffic pollution.

DEFICIENCY SYMPTOMS OF VITAMIN C

The classic vitamin-C deficiency disease of scurvy manifests itself as bleeding of the gums, loosening of the teeth, lassitude, weakness, irritability, and aching muscles. Nowadays, deficiency tends to be marginal but occurs over a prolonged period of time and may predispose toward cancer and heart disease.

VITAMIN C SUPPLEMENTATION

Vitamin C is not toxic, though excessive intake may cause diarrhea. However, the level of bowel tolerance can vary greatly between individuals. In some, taking 10g a day of vitamin C will not cause diarrhea, whereas in others as little as 500mg a day may do so. Vitamin C is available in many forms—powders, crystals, capsules, tablets, timed-release—and the actual amount of vitamin C varies considerably. Ascorbic acid is the most widely used and least expensive, but can sometimes be irritating to the digestive system. "Buffered" preparations are less harsh and are combined with different minerals—sodium, magnesium, calcium, or potassium—though sodium ascorbate may be a problem where sodium sensitivity exists. Much of the vitamin C in supplements is derived from corn, but for individuals who are sensitive to this grain, the sago palm is an additional source.

Research has indicated that a dose of around 1,000mg (1g) to 3,000mg (3g) per day can be maintained safely, with higher doses being used for short duration to ward off colds or treat infections. However, make sure that your daily intake is no more than 1,000mg if you are taking the contraceptive pill, since estrogen and vitamin C share the same excretory pathway; estrogens will remain in the body at a higher level, turning a low-dose pill into a high-dose one. Also, excessive intake over long periods of time can interfere with the absorption of other

RIGHT Supplements come in a variety of forms—choose the one that suits you.

RIGHT Snack on raspberries or strawberries for a tasty vitamin C boost.

nutrients; ensure that your high vitamin C dose is taken at a time distant from intake of food and other supplements. The results of blood and urine tests can be altered by the presence of large amounts of vitamin C, so let your physician know if you are supplementing your diet with vitamin C. When cutting down from a large dose to a smaller dose of vitamin C, do this gradually so that "rebound" deficiency symptoms do not occur. To increase the absorption rate of vitamin C, bioflavonoids, calcium, and magnesium are needed. Also, since vitamin C is intricately involved with other nutritional antioxidants—including beta-carotene, vitamin E, and selenium—a combination of antioxidants may provide greater benefit than any single nutrient.

There is no known adverse interaction with vitamin C and any drug, though vitamin C may possibly dilute the effect of tricyclic antidepressants (for example, amitriptyline and imipramine). There are no contraindications for its use, especially at low to moderate levels.

MARGINAL DEFICIENCY SYMPTOMS

WEAKNESS

POOR HEALING OF WOUNDS

EASY BRUISING

JOINT PAIN

SLOW RECOVERY FROM COLDS AND FLU

BLEEDING, SORE GUMS

FATIGUE

HYPOGLYCEMIA

SKIN PROBLEMS

RIGHT Vitamin C is traditionally used to treat the symptoms of colds and flu.

CLINICAL REPORT

Cancer prevention Cervical cancer risk is increased dramatically with low vitamin C intake. Some research indicates that women with intakes less than 88mg per day have a fourfold increase. Those women with cervical dysplasia, which is often seen as a precancerous condition, appear to have a significantly low intake of vitamin C and low blood levels of the vitamin compared with women with normal cervixes.

Cholesterol reduction Much clinical and observational research work shows that vitamin C levels correspond to cholesterol levels. One piece of work in particular indicated that the higher the vitamin C content of the blood, the lower the total cholesterol and triglycerides and the higher the HDL cholesterol ("good" cholesterol). Even small rises in vitamin C content in the blood appeared to correlate with increased levels of HDL cholesterol. This study, among others, demonstrates that the relationship between vitamin C and HDL cholesterol persists even where well-nourished individuals (with normal levels of vitamin C in their blood) supplement their diets with additional vitamin C. However, there does seem to be a threshold level after which increasing vitamin C intake shows no further improvement. Some work indicates that this threshold level may be around 200mg per day for women and 350mg per day for men. This, of course, is good news; it means that large doses of vitamin C, which may cause diarrhea, are not necessary to obtain the protective effect of high HDL cholesterol levels.

VITAMIN D

Vitamin D is produced in the body by the action of sunlight on the skin. For this reason, many scientists consider it more of a hormone than a vitamin. It is found in foods mainly of animal origin and was isolated in 1930 from cod liver oil. There are two main forms of this vitamin, namely vitamin D2 and vitamin D3. It is vitamin D3 (cholecalciferol) which is made by the action of sunlight on cholesterol deposits in the skin. Because of this, is it often referred to as the "sunshine vitamin." It is also found in animal liver oils, since the liver is where vitamin D is stored.

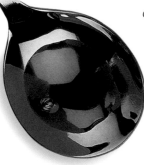

ABOVE A convenient to take vitamin D.

LEFT Cod liver oil is rich in vitamin D.

Vitamin D2 (ergocalciferol) is the plant form of the vitamin formed by the action of ultraviolet light on ergosterol in the plant. Vitamin D is a fat-soluble nutrient and is the only vitamin required in greater quantities by children than adults, for the very reason that it is needed for the absorption of calcium and phosphorus from the gut to enable proper growth of healthy bones.

Deficiency of vitamin D in childhood leads to the development of the deficiency disease rickets. This disease may show itself as early as two months of age when areas of softening on the skull are observed. Development of teeth may be delayed and the posture greatly affected. Characteristically, it causes the bowing of the legs when a child starts to walk. In adults, severe vitamin D deficiency presents as osteomalacia. Since bones have stopped growing, the symptoms are different. Osteomalacia usually occurs as thinning and weakening of the bone and spontaneous fractures may occur. Nowadays, however, rickets and osteomalacia are not very common in developed countries, especially as multivitamin drops for babies and children are so widely used.

These diseases may continue to be found in ethnic communities where there is a tendency to cover most of the body, preventing vitamin D being made by sunlight, and where the cultural diet dictates very little in the way of high vitamin D foods.

DIETARY REFERENCE VALUES FOR VITAMIN D

	mcg/day	rni IU/day	rda IU/day
0–6 MONTHS	8.5	340	300
7 MONTHS TO 3 YEARS	7	280	400
4–10 YEARS	0*	0*	400
11–24 YEARS	0*	0*	400
25–64 YEARS	0*	0*	200
65 + YEARS	10	400	200
PREGNANCY	10	400	400
LACTATION	10	400	400

*It is assumed that in the 4–64 year age group, vitamin D formed by the exposure of skin to sunlight is satisfactory for daily needs.

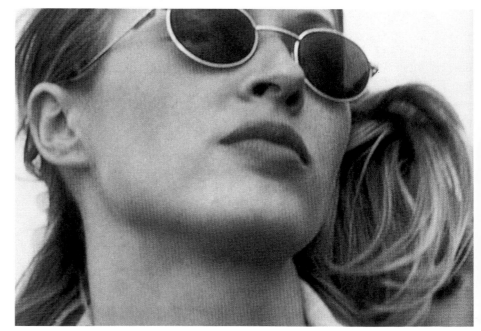

LEFT Vitamin D is formed by the action of sunlight on the skin.

DIETARY SOURCES OF VITAMIN D		
	mcg/100g	IU/100g
COD LIVER OIL	212.5	8,500
HERRING AND KIPPER	22.4	896
SALMON, CANNED	12.5	500
EGGS	1.6	64
BUTTER	0.8	32
LIVER	0.8	32
CHEESE, CHEDDAR	0.3	12
MILK, WHOLE	0.03	1.2
DARK GREEN LEAFY VEGETABLES	TRACE	TRACE
SHIITAKE MUSHROOMS	TRACE	TRACE

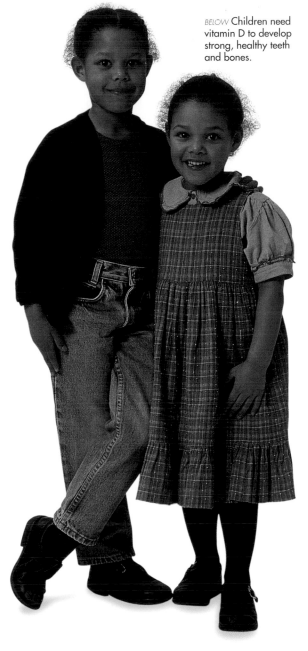

BELOW Children need vitamin D to develop strong, healthy teeth and bones.

VITAMIN D CONTENT IN FOOD

There are very few independent dietary sources of vitamin D. Fatty fish such as herring, mackerel, salmon, pilchards, sardines, and tuna are rich sources, but are not, generally, major contributors to the diet. The only other useful sources are eggs and fortified foods including margarine (which is required to contain vitamin D by law), some yogurts and breakfast cereals. The amount of vitamin D in meat is uncertain. Vegetables are low in vitamin D, but the best sources are dark green leafy vegetables and mushrooms. Vitamin D is stored in the body and is replenished by the activity of sunlight on the skin.

FUNCTIONS OF VITAMIN D

Vitamin D is best known for its ability to stimulate calcium absorption. In the skin, sunlight changes the vitamin D precursor into cholecalciferol (D3). This is then transported to the liver and converted to a compound, which is five times more potent than D3. This derivative of vitamin D3 is then converted in the kidneys into yet another substance, which is ten times more potent than D3. Therefore, disorders of the liver or kidneys result in impaired conversion of vitamin D and, ultimately, poor absorption of calcium. Many patients with osteoporosis have high levels of the liver intermediary, but low levels of the kidney form of vitamin D, which indicates that impairment in kidney conversion reactions is a factor in osteoporosis. There is some evidence that suggests estrogen, magnesium, and the mineral boron are all involved in this conversion reaction.

FUNCTIONS OF VITAMIN D

• Necessary for the absorption of calcium, phosphorus, magnesium, zinc, iron, and other minerals.

• Important for healthy formation of bones and teeth.

• Involved in the metabolism of calcium and phosphorus.

• Increases excretion of phosphorus from the kidneys.

• Helps the body utilize vitamin A.

• Required for kidney function.

• Anticancer activity, especially against breast and colon cancer.

• Used therapeutically to help osteoporosis and other bone diseases, psoriasis, deafness, prevention of colds, conjunctivitis, and migraine.

LEFT **Kippers are among the highest sources of vitamin D.**

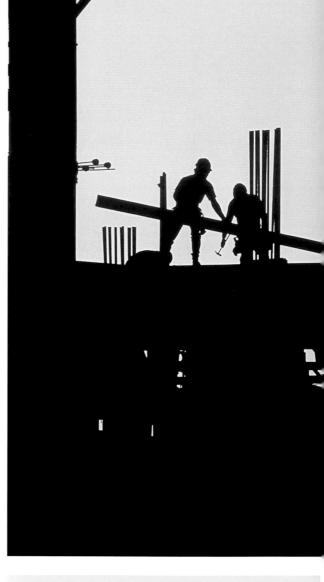

RIGHT **Nightworkers who rarely see the sun may need a vitamin D supplement.**

VITAMIN D SUPPLEMENTATION

Generally vitamin D, as cholecalciferol or vitamin D3, is supplemented as part of a multivitamin complex. Most capsules contain approximately 400IU (in the form of natural fish-liver oils) and doses of between 250 and 1,000IU can be taken daily. The most common form of supplementation is natural cod-liver oil in either capsule or oil form.

Supplementation may be useful for:
• Nightworkers.
• Those living in highly polluted areas.
• Elderly people, particularly those who are housebound.
• Those wearing traditional dress which covers most of the body.
• Vegans, especially those living in cold climates.
• Lactating women, whose breastmilk can be low in vitamin D, especially in winter months.

CLINICAL REPORT

Anecdotal evidence from a small group of women with a history of menstrual-related migraines indicates that supplementation with a combination of vitamin D and calcium resulted in a major reduction in headaches and premenstrual symptoms within two months of beginning therapy. However, since vitamin D facilitates the absorption of several minerals, including calcium, magnesium, iron, and zinc, it is very likely that it is the generalized increased availability of minerals that helps with migraine and menstrual problems.

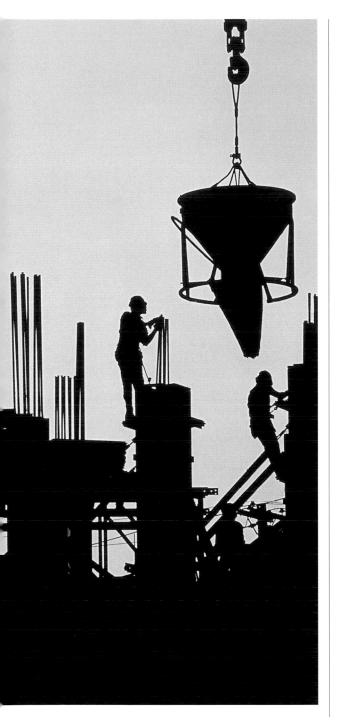

RICKETS IN CHILDREN	OSTEOPOROSIS
OSTEOMALACIA	TOOTH DECAY
BONE PAIN	PREMATURE AGING
MUSCULAR WEAKNESS AND SPASM	LACK OF SUNLIGHT

Some researchers suggest that long-term overconsumption of vitamin D (or calcium) in fortified foods may contribute to athero-sclerosis and heart disease, possibly as a result of a decrease in magnesium absorption or because of some form of calcium deposition in the blood vessels.

When digitoxin and certain other cardiac glycoside heart drugs are taken in combination with vitamin D, there is a slight risk that abnormal heart rhythm may occur.

ABOVE Fresh shiitake mushrooms contain a trace of vitamin D.

The drugs cholestyramine, Dilantin, and phenobarbital and mineral oil all interfere with the absorption and/or metabolism of vitamin D.

TOXICITY

Vitamin D is the most toxic of all the vitamins because of its fat-solubility and ability to reach very high levels in the body, a state leading to hypercalcemia. Symptoms of toxicity may include nausea, vomiting, headache, depression, unusual thirst, sore eyes, and pruritus (itching). High levels of vitamin D in the body may lead to damage to the arteries, kidney stones, irregular heartbeat, high blood pressure, and calcium "dumping" (calcium deposited inappropriately in soft tissues). In adults, symptoms of vitamin D toxicity have been reported at daily intakes of 625mcg (25,000IU). Doses in excess of 1,000IU daily are not recommended unless under the supervision of a registered practitioner.

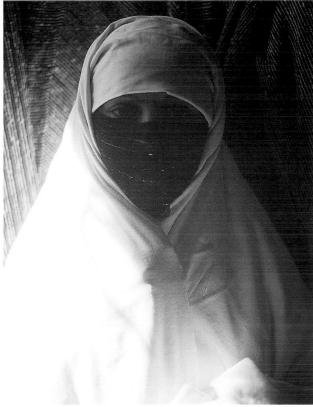

ABOVE People who wear traditional dress, covering the body from top to toe, may require vitamin D supplementation.

VITAMIN E

Vitamin E is a fat-soluble nutrient consisting of four substances—alpha, beta, delta, and gamma tocopherol. It was originally discovered to be a fertility factor in animals—the word "tocopherol" comes from the Greek tokos *meaning "offspring" and* phero *meaning "to bear." There are natural and synthetic forms of all the tocopherols, but the naturally occurring form of vitamin E is in the alpha group and is the "D" form, as in D-alpha tocopherol (the synthetic form is DL-alpha tocopherol). D-alpha tocopherol is much more absorbable than other forms. It is an antioxidant vitamin with a wide range of therapeutic uses. Despite being fat-soluble, vitamin E is stored less efficiently by the body than most other fat-soluble nutrients and up to 70 percent of intake is excreted in the feces each day. It is stored in the liver, fatty tissues, heart, testes, uterus, muscles, blood, and the adrenal and pituitary glands.*

ABOVE Fresh, raw sunflower seeds are a rich source of vitamin E.

white blood cell

cancerous

ABOVE Vitamin E, taken in high doses, may protect against cancer.

Most animal species, including man, require vitamin E. In 1922, researchers discovered that rats became infertile when they ate a purified diet lacking in vitamin E. When oils containing vitamin E were added to their diet, their ability to reproduce returned.

Vitamin E functions primarily as an antioxidant in protecting against free radical damage to cell membranes. It is the foremost "lipid phase" antioxidant in the body, meaning that it is actually incorporated into the lipid (fatty) part of the cell membranes. In this position, it acts to stabilize and protect these structures from heavy metals such as lead and mercury; toxic materials like benzene, carbon tetrachloride, and cleaning solvents; drugs; radiation; and the body's own free-radical metabolites, plus those from overprocessed and burned food. Because of these antioxidant activities, a high vitamin E diet is important, particularly in protecting the immune system during times of oxidative stress from damaging viral illnesses such as AIDS and chronic viral hepatitis. Additionally, vitamin E has been found to be more effective than many of the anticoagulant drugs used in cardiovascular disease and has an excellent safety profile

at high intake, unlike the other fat-soluble vitamins A (retinol) and vitamin D.

No less important is vitamin E's role in protecting against heart disease, stroke, and cancer. Like other antioxidants, such as vitamin A and beta-carotene, vitamin E offers much protection against cancer when taken in high doses. Many studies have shown that low vitamin-E levels (especially when combined with low selenium levels) increase the risk of certain types of cancer, particularly those of the gastrointestinal tract and lung. One study showed that individuals with a low blood level of vitamin E had a 50 percent greater risk of developing cancer than those with high levels.

Diabetics appear to have an increased requirement for vitamin E. This is probably due to the fact that oxidative stress is a major factor in diabetes. Vitamin E is able to improve insulin action and its antioxidant properties are likely to prevent some of the long-term complications of diabetes such as cardiovascular disease, kidney damage, nerve degeneration, and eye problems.

DIETARY REFERENCE VALUES FOR VITAMIN E		
	rda mg/day	rda IU/day
1–10 YEARS	6–7	9–10.5
ADULTS	10	15
PREGNANCY	10	15
LACTATION	12	18

DIETARY SOURCES OF VITAMIN E MG/100G

WHEAT-GERM OIL	178	SPINACH	2.7
SUNFLOWER SEEDS, FRESH AND RAW	97	BROCCOLI FLORETS, RAW	2.0
SUNFLOWER OIL	74	CORNMEAL, UNENRICHED, COOKED	1.52
ALMONDS, FRESH, WHOLE	37	BLACKCURRANTS, RAW	1.32
HAZELNUTS, FRESH, WHOLE	28	PECANS, UNSALTED	1.30
MAYONNAISE	19	CANTALOUPE, RAW	1.08
WHEAT-GERM	17	CHESTNUTS, FRESH	1.00
PEANUTS, RAW WITH SKINS	15	BEANS, WHITE, COOKED	0.94
PEANUT BUTTER	9	COCONUT, FRESH, GRATED	0.91
BRAZIL NUTS, FRESH, WHOLE	9	PEAS, GARDEN, COOKED	0.83
SOY OIL	8	BEETGREENS	0.57
TURNIP GREENS	5	WALNUTS, FRESH	0.48
BLACKBERRIES	5	CELERY, RAW	0.46
OATS, ROLLED (OATMEAL), COOKED	5	CARROTS, RAW	0.45
SWEET POTATO, ALL VARIETIES, RAW	4	BANANAS	0.3
RYE, WHOLE-GRAIN	3	STRAWBERRIES	0.3
BUTTER	3	RED CABBAGE	0.22
ASPARAGUS	2.7		

BELOW Eating plenty of raw foods, particularly vegetables, can boost your intake of vitamin E.

All in all, vitamin E appears to be a crucial preventative factor against the Western world's three leading killer diseases—heart disease, cancer, and stroke.

DIETARY REFERENCE VALUES FOR VITAMIN E

The requirement for vitamin E is related to the polyunsaturated fatty acid (PUFA) content of the diet. Also, individual people's requirements are thought to vary greatly. It is considered that, since PUFA intakes vary so widely, it is not possible to set strict guidelines. There are, therefore, no RNIs set for vitamin E. If an average intake of PUFA is considered to provide around six percent of dietary energy, then for males 18–50 years old, intake of vitamin E would be around 7mg/day, and for females of 18–50 years the figure should be around 5mg/day. However, a level of 0.4mg vitamin E per gram of dietary PUFA has been presumed adequate in American diets. There are RDA figures for vitamin E (*see* opposite).

VITAMIN E CONTENT IN FOOD

The amount of vitamin E required is largely dependent upon the amount of polyunsaturated fats (PUFAs) in the diet. It is a vitamin that is generally very easily absorbed in the digestive tract. The variability in absorption rate in different individuals is likely to reflect the health of the intestinal lining in these people.

The more polyunsaturated fats are consumed, the greater the risk that they will be damaged by oxidation. Since vitamin E prevents this damage, as the intake of PUFAs increases, so does the need for vitamin E to protect the essential fatty acids from free radical damage (oxidation). Fortunately, where there are high levels of PUFAs, there are also higher levels of vitamin E. Nature ensures that important PUFAs are protected. The best sources of vitamin E are fresh nuts and seeds and their oils, soybeans, and some whole grains. A fairly wide range of fruits and vegetables, especially berries, asparagus, sweet potatoes, and green leafy vegetables also contain vitamin E in reasonable amounts.

Vitamin E is extremely vulnerable to processing. It is destroyed by heat, oxygen, freezing, and chlorine found in drinking water. Vegetables that have been frozen for longer than two months are likely to have very little vitamin E content left in them.

Smokers and women taking the contraceptive pill will need extra vitamin E, since both cigarette smoke and excess estrogens are likely to deplete the body of its vitamin E reserves. Pregnant and breastfeeding women usually have a higher requirement for vitamin E.

Vitamin E interacts extensively with other antioxidant nutrients, especially vitamin C and selenium. It also improves the action of vitamin A and helps convert vitamin B12 to its active form. This is good evidence to show that a healthy diet should contain a wide range of fresh produce to help maximize this synergistic effect that many nutrients appear to have, one with another.

FUNCTIONS OF VITAMIN E

Vitamin E is a prime antioxidant and is especially important for prevention of oxidative damage to foods high in polyunsaturated fatty acids and to lipid-containing structures within the body. This means that all cells depend upon vitamin E to preserve the integrity of their membranes, including those of the reproductive system. Vitamin E is particularly important in immune function. In addition to protecting the thymus gland and circulating white blood cells from damage, vitamin E is especially important for protecting and strengthening the immune system, while it is excellent for fighting chronic viral illnesses like AIDS and hepatitis.

The antioxidant protection of vitamin E is also obviously needed for a healthy nervous system and to prevent premature degeneration of nerves and muscles. Children and adults who are unable to absorb or utilize vitamin E adequately can develop a characteristic and progressive neurological syndrome involving the central and peripheral nervous system, retina, and skeletal muscles. Additionally, vitamin E is able to reduce the oxygen requirement of muscles and thereby increase exercise capacity. It is protective against atherosclerosis and thrombosis and is often found to be better at preventing blood clots than more conventional anticoagulant medications.

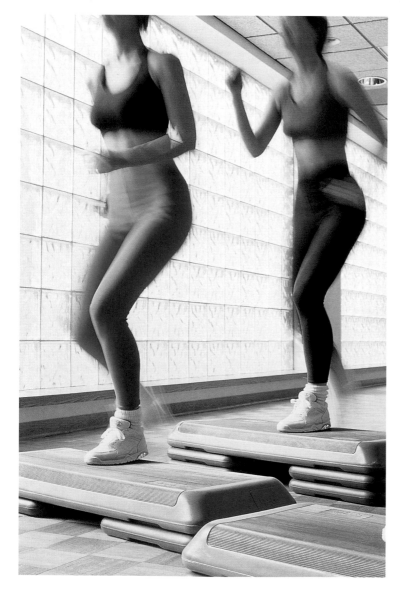

LEFT Vitamin E is able to redefine the oxygen requirement of muscles and increase exercise capacity.

FUNCTIONS OF VITAMIN E

- Antioxidant.
- Necessary for healthy immune function.
- Slows aging process.
- Protects against pollution.
- Helps develop and maintain nerves and muscles.

- Reduces oxygen requirements of muscles.
- Helps prevent miscarriages.
- Works as a natural diuretic.
- Prevents scarring of the skin (when applied topically).
- Improves fertility.

ABOVE **Dark green, leafy vegetables, such as spinach, are a valuable source of this important vitamin.**

DEFICIENCY SYMPTOMS

Deficiency of vitamin E does not lead to any specific disease state in the short term, but long term insufficiency is thought to be a contributing factor in cancer and heart disease. In children, fat malabsorption may cause a deficiency of vitamin E and can lead to the development of abnormal red blood cells. Anyone with heart problems (atherosclerosis, angina, thrombosis, or elevated cholesterol), cancer, cataracts, circulatory disorders, fibrocystic breast disease, increased blood platelet coagulation, or Parkinson's disease may be suffering, at least in part, from borderline deficiency in this vitamin.

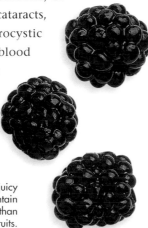

RIGHT **Fresh, juicy blackberries contain more vitamin E than many other fruits.**

USED THERAPEUTICALLY TO HELP TREATMENT OF:

VARICOSE VEINS	INFERTILITY
COLD SORES AND OTHER SKIN PROBLEMS	IMPOTENCE
MENOPAUSAL PROBLEMS	SOME ANEMIAS
AGE SPOTS	CATARACTS
PMS	FRAGILE RED BLOOD CELLS
MUSCLE DEGENERATION	

USED THERAPEUTICALLY TO HELP TREATMENT OF:

ACNE	CAPILLARY FRAGILITY	INTERMITTENT CLAUDICATION	PEPTIC ULCERS
AIDS	CATARACT	LUPUS	PERIODONTAL DISEASE
ALCOHOL-INDUCED LIVER DISEASE	CERVICAL DYSPLASIA	MACULAR DEGENERATION	PMS
ALLERGY	DIABETES	MENOPAUSAL SYMPTOMS	RAYNAUD'S DISEASE
ANEMIA	ECZEMA	MULTIPLE SCLEROSIS	RHEUMATOID ARTHRITIS
ANGINA	EPILEPSY	NEURALGIA	SCLERODERMA
ATHEROSCLEROSIS	GALLSTONES	NEUROMUSCULAR DEGENERATION	SEBORRHEIC DERMATITIS
AUTOIMMUNE DISORDERS	GANGRENE	OSTEOARTHRITIS	SKIN ULCERS
BURNS	HEPATITIS	PARKINSON'S DISEASE	ULCERATIVE COLITIS
CANCER	HERPES INFECTIONS		WOUND HEALING
	INFLAMMATION		

VITAMIN E SUPPLEMENTATION

Vitamin E is available in many forms, but the most active is natural D-alpha tocopherol. It is usually taken as an oil (in capsules), though dried (powder) capsules are available. Dosages of between 200 and 300IU (134–201mg) per day are usually considered adequate, although smokers, pregnant and breastfeeding women, and women of menopausal age will require more. Therapeutically, vitamin E can be safely taken in doses up to 1,000IU (671mg) per day. Since vitamin E and selenium work synergistically, for every 200IU (134mg) vitamin E, take 25mcg of selenium to encourage the efficiency of the vitamin.

Vitamin E is thought to be safe up to levels of around 4,0768IU (3,200mg) per day, though a daily intake of around 800IU (537mg) D-alpha tocopherol (active vitamin E) has occasionally been associated with such symptoms as fatigue, nausea, mild gastrointestinal problems, palpitations, and transient blood pressure increase. Such symptoms are, however, reversible and to minimize their onset, larger doses can be achieved by gradually increasing the amount over several weeks. However, those people suffering from high blood pressure should discuss vitamin E supplementation with their practitioner beforehand. Because of vitamin E's ability to reduce coagulation of the blood, it should be taken only under medical supervision by people already taking anti-

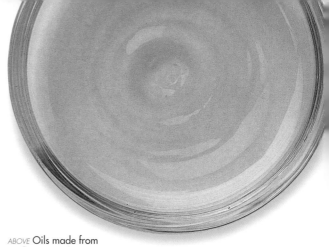

ABOVE Oils made from sunflower seeds, sesame seeds, soya, and nuts are very high in vitamin E.

coagulant medication. Similarly, diabetics and people who suffer from hypothyroidism should avoid high intake levels of supplementary vitamin E unless under the supervision of a practitioner. There is also some concern with the taking of large doses of vitamin E by women who are receiving medication for breast cancer. If in doubt, discuss your requirements with your general physician before taking any additional vitamin E.

Inorganic iron, in the form of ferrous sulfate, destroys vitamin E activity and should not, therefore, be taken within eight hours of taking vitamin E. A better choice to take would be an organic form of iron such as iron ascorbate malate.

BELOW A selection of fresh vegetables will provide plenty of vitamin E.

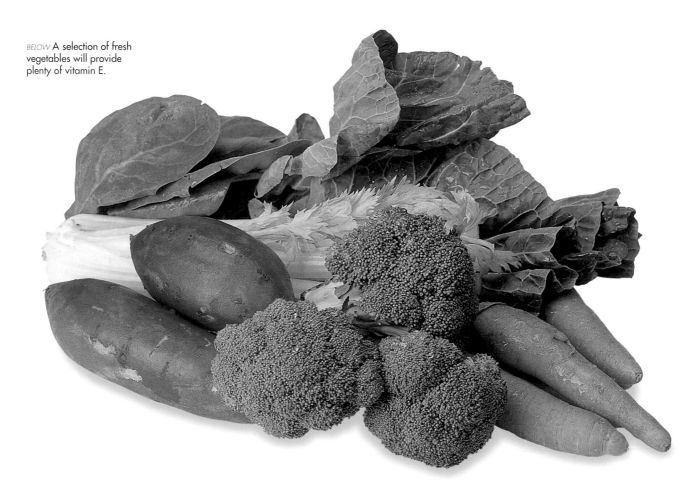

CLINICAL REPORTS

HEART DISEASE AND STROKE

Confirmed anti-antherosclerotic effects of vitamin E include an ability to reduce LDL cholesterol ("bad" cholesterol), increase HDL cholesterol ("good" cholesterol), and inhibit excessive blood platelet aggregation. Much research has demonstrated that vitamin E status may be more predictive of developing a heart attack or stroke than total cholesterol levels. One particular study has shown that low blood levels of vitamin E was a predictive factor for heart attack in approximately three times more cases than either high blood cholesterol or high blood pressure. Dosages of around 400 to 800IU (268–537mg) per day seem to be the protective range, with lower doses not being so effective.

Since nut and seed oils are high in vitamin E, this may be the reason why the Mediterranean diet, with its copious olive oil, is so protective of the heart. It might also be part of the answer to the "French paradox"—a large amount of fatty food is eaten in France, yet heart disease is lower than in Britain or America. The essential factor in both of these cases has been attributed to red wine and its high level of protective anthocyanidins, but vitamin E in the diet is also likely to be a contributing factor.

FIBROCYSTIC BREAST DISEASE

Fibrocystic breast disease can be a mildly uncomfortable swelling of the breast, but is often severely painful. It typically occurs in cycles and usually precedes a period. In many women it is a component in PMS. It is thought to affect 20 to 40 percent of premenopausal women and is considered a risk for developing breast cancer.

Several double-blind studies have indicated that vitamin E, as alphatocopherol, relieves many PMS components but in particular breast pain. The exact reason for this is still not fully known, but it may be that vitamin E at around 600IU (402mg) per day normalizes female hormone levels.

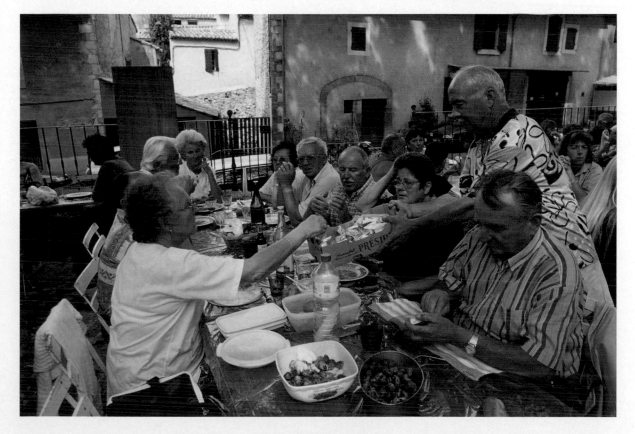

ABOVE The Mediterranean
diet, rich in vitamin E,
protects the heart.

VITAMIN K

Vitamin K is an important fat-soluble vitamin, stored in the bones and the liver. Chemically, phylloquinone is the natural plant source of vitamin K, but a synthetic derivative, menadione, is used therapeutically. Vitamin K treats specific deficiencies that occur during anticoagulant therapy and in hemorrhagic diseases of the newborn. Although the body stores very little vitamin K, it is rarely deficient.

LEFT Vitamin K is found in a variety of vegetables, especially string beans.

In a healthy gut, the beneficial bacteria produce vitamin K compounds, called menaquinones. Thus, a high dietary intake is not as crucial as it is for other vitamins. Nevertheless, it does mean that a healthy digestive tract is essential for the correct balance of bacterial species. Taking live yogurt (dairy or soy) daily will encourage the growth of these useful organisms. The main function of vitamin K is to aid in the complex mechanism of blood clotting. Recent research is showing that vitamin K is also involved in bone metabolism; specifically it is needed for correct formation of the bone protein, osteocalcin, which is the protein holding calcium in place in the bones. It may be essential in the prevention and treatment of osteoporosis.

Vitamin K's primary role is in the manufacture of clotting factors in the liver, where the various forms of vitamin K appear to function similarly. However, in other roles—for example, the production of osteocalcin—the phylloquinone form would appear to be superior.

DIETARY REFERENCE VALUES (DRV) FOR VITAMIN K

The range of adult vitamin K requirements for RNIs is not yet known, but 1mcg per kilogram of body weight per day (around 60mcg per day for an average adult) is considered safe and adequate since it maintains vitamin K-dependent clotting factors at normal concentrations and in their active form. The requirement for babies is based on a DRV for breast milk that, for infants consuming 1½ pints (850ml), would be around 8.5mcg phylloquinone per day, rounded up to a safe intake of 10mcg per day to make allowances for the low concentrations of menaquinones from gut bacteria at this stage in life. American RDAs give 20mcg/day for a child aged 4–6 years, 30–45mcg/day for children aged 7–14 years, and between 60 and 80mcg/day for adults.

VITAMIN K CONTENT OF FOOD

The predominant dietary form of vitamin K is phylloquinone, found in the highest amounts in dark green leafy vegetables; asparagus, oats, whole wheat, and fresh green peas are also good sources. Significant amounts can be found in other vegetables, kelp, fruits, vegetable oils, egg yolks, liver, fish liver oils, and meats. Because of healthy bacterial activity, live yogurt is also a useful source. An intact and healthy gut with a good balance of appropriate bacteria will provide the menaquinones.

About 70 percent of dietary vitamin K is regularly excreted, so a healthy digestive system, together with a good daily intake of high vitamin K foods is needed for healthy blood clotting.

FUNCTIONS OF VITAMIN K

- Vital for the formation of blood-clotting factors.

- Involved in the formation of bone proteins and appropriate calcification of bone.

- Prevention of osteoporosis.

- Used to help in the treatment of excessive menstrual bleeding.

- Used therapeutically in hemorrhagic disease of the newborn.

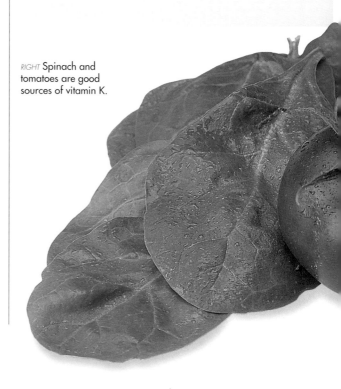

RIGHT Spinach and tomatoes are good sources of vitamin K.

DIETARY SOURCES OF VITAMIN K (MCG/100G)	
CAULIFLOWER, RAW	3,600
BRUSSELS SPROUTS, RAW	1,888
KALE	729
GREEN TEA	712
TURNIP GREENS	650
SPINACH	415
TOMATOES	400
RUNNER BEANS	290
BROCCOLI	200
SOYBEANS, COOKED	190
LETTUCE	129
CABBAGE	125
POTATOES, BOILED	80
WATERCRESS	57
ASPARAGUS, BOILED	57
HARD CHEESE	50
MEAT, COOKED	50
OATS	20
GREEN PEAS	19
WHOLE WHEAT	17

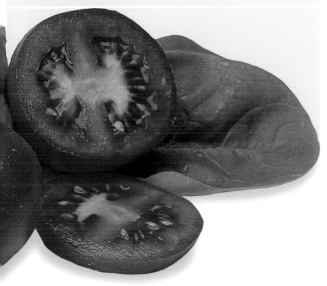

CLINICAL REPORT

A deficiency of vitamin K (phylloquinone) may lead to impaired mineralization of bone because of inadequate osteocalcin levels. Patients with fractures due to the presence of osteoporitic bone usually exhibit very low blood levels of vitamin K. Some clinical research has demonstrated a correlation between the severity of fracture and circulating blood levels of vitamin K, with the lower levels of the vitamin showing the greatest severity of fracture.

SUPPLEMENTATION OF VITAMIN K

The vitamin is not routinely supplemented except for newborn babies. However, supplements are used therapeutically in the prevention of internal bleeding, excessive menstrual bleeding, and in treating deficiencies that occur during anticoagulant therapy. More than 500mcg of synthetic vitamin K (menadione) for an adult is not recommended.

Vitamin K administration may counteract the anti-coagulant actions of drugs like warfarin and coumadin. These drugs work to prevent clot formation by blocking the activity of vitamin K. Aspirin, certain antibiotics, and high doses of vitamin E (greater than 600IU per day) also antagonize vitamin K action. Otherwise, there are no known side effects or toxicity.

Adequate amounts can be obtained from food for most deficiencies; increase your dietary intake of cauliflower and other green leafy vegetables. Alternatively, take it as part of a multiformula with a level around 20mcg per tablet.

DEFICIENCY SYMPTOMS	
OSTEOPOROSIS	FAT MALABSORPTION (PREVENTION OF ABSORPTION)
EXCESSIVE MENSTRUAL BLEEDING	
POOR BLOOD-CLOTTING AFTER INJURY	DRAMATIC REDUCTION OF HEALTHY BACTERIA IN THE GUT (CAUSED BY EXTENDED COURSES OF ANTIBIOTICS)
FREQUENT NOSEBLEEDS	
CHRONIC DIARRHEA (PREVENTION OF ABSORPTION AND LOW BACTERIAL LEVELS)	DISEASES OF THE DIGESTIVE TRACT (IMBALANCE OF HEALTHY BACTERIA AND POOR ABSORPTION)

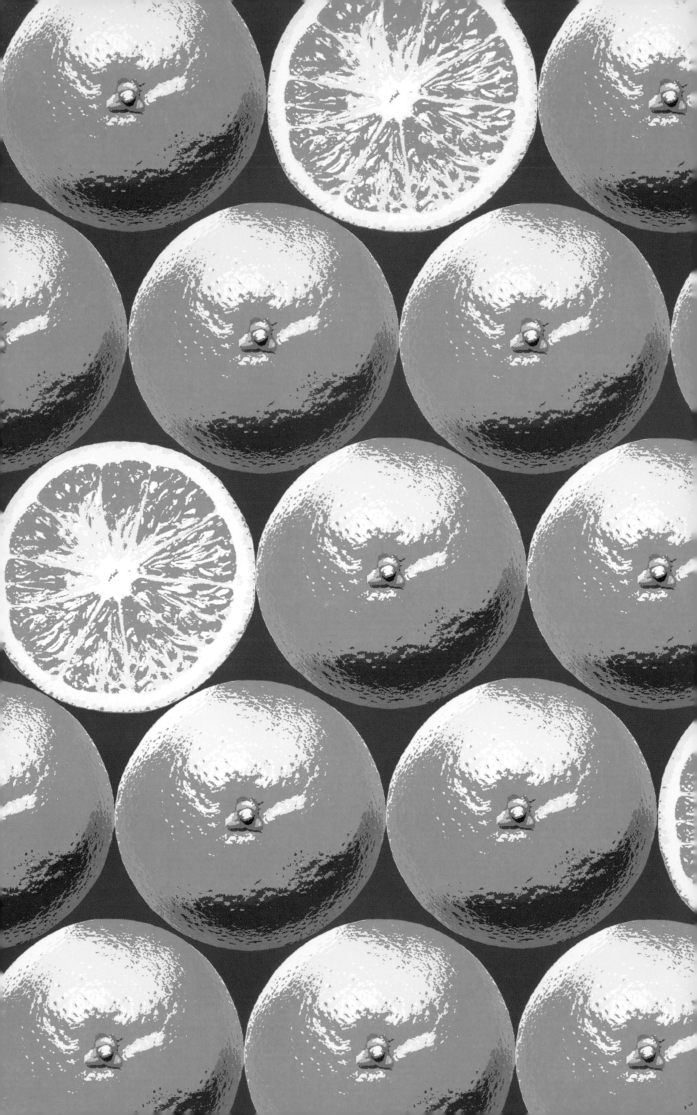

PART THREE

THE MINERALS

Minerals are basically metals and other inorganic compounds that work within the body in much the same way as vitamins, promoting body processes and providing much of the structure for teeth and bones. Minerals are classified in two groups. Proper, or major minerals, are needed in quantities of over 100mg per day; these include calcium, phosphorus, potassium, sodium, chloride, magnesium, and sulfer. Minor minerals, or trace elements, are required by the body in quantities less than 100mg per day, and include chromium, zinc, selenium, silicon, boron, copper, manganese, molybdemum, and vanadium. In this section, the most important minerals are listed, along with their function, and the recommended dosage of each supplement is also given.

CALCIUM

Calcium is the most abundant mineral in the human body, comprising over 1.5 percent of the total body weight. Of the 2lb12oz (1.25kg) of calcium in the body, approximately 99 percent of this calcium is found in the bones and teeth, with the remaining one percent in the soft tissues, blood, and tissue fluid. Absorption of calcium is intimately associated with, and dependent upon, vitamin D. Deficiencies of vitamin D and calcium are often, therefore, related.

ABOVE Mouth-watering olives—a good source of calcium.

ABOVE Shrimp are among the seafoods that contain calcium.

Transmission of nervous impulses along nerves, the release of neuro-transmitters, and the contraction of muscle, including heart muscle and smooth (involuntary) muscle, depend on calcium. It is essential for many enzyme reactions, both inside and outside cells, as well as general cellular structure, and is an essential component of the blood clotting mechanism. Recent research indicates that modern diets contain only around one-third of the calcium needed.

Young growing children are able to absorb a higher proportion of dietary calcium than adults. In adults, women are more often calcium-deficient than men and, in the elderly (especially elderly women), deficiency can be considerable. Some individuals can adapt to a prolonged low intake by increasing the efficiency of absorption, though an intact, healthy digestive lining is required.

For most people in the Western world, the primary source of calcium is dairy products (and especially cow's milk). However, it is a mistake to assume that dairy products are the best source of calcium. Calcium is present in an extremely wide range of foods, many of which contain it in far higher quantities than milk. These alternative sources are, on the whole more nutritionally balanced than milk, which has high calcium and saturated fat, but is poor in magnesium and iron. Moreover, although Cheddar cheese is an extremely calcium-rich food, it is also very high in saturated fat and very low in magnesium. Calcium and magnesium are minerals that work in tandem in a healthy body and a dietary excess of one will mean a consequent reduction in the level of the other, leading to imbalance.

Therefore, it is far better to obtain your calcium from vegetarian foods like bean curd, dark green vegetables, and nuts and seeds which are high in both calcium and magnesium. Furthermore, the fats in nuts and seeds contain essential polyunsaturated fatty acids in large amounts. These are vital for healthy nerve, immune, hormonal, and brain function.

DIETARY REFERENCE VALUES FOR CALCIUM		
	rni mg/day	rda mg/day
0–12 MONTHS	525	400–600
1–3 YEARS	350	800
4–6 YEARS	450	800
7–10 YEARS	550	800
11–18 YEARS (MALES)	1,000	
11–24 (MALES)		1,200
11–18 YEARS (FEMALES)	800	
11–24 (FEMALES)		1,200
19+ YEARS	700	
24+ YEARS		800
PREGNANCY	700	1,200
LACTATION	1,250	1,200

BELOW Dandelion leaves, an unusual way to take calcium.

DIETARY SOURCES OF CALCIUM MG/100G					
KELP	1,093	DANDELION LEAVES	187	ROMAINE LETTUCE	68
CHEESE, CHEDDAR	750	BRAZIL NUTS	186	APRICOTS, DRIED	67
SESAME SEEDS	700	GOAT'S MILK	129	PEANUTS, ROASTED	61
SARDINES, WITH (SOFT) BONES	550	SHRIMP, COOKED	125	BLACKCURRANTS	60
BEAN CURD	506	SUNFLOWER SEEDS	120	CABBAGE	57
MOLASSES	450	BUCKWHEAT, RAW	114	BREAD, WHOLE-WHEAT	54
CAROB FLOUR	352	OLIVES, RIPE	106	BOSTON BAKED BEANS	53
PULSES	296	PILCHARDS, WITH (SOFT) BONES	105	EGGS	52
FIGS, DRIED	280	BROCCOLI	103	GLOBE ARTICHOKE	51
KALE	249	MILK, WHOLE	103	PUMPKIN SEEDS	51
TURNIP GREENS	246	WALNUTS	99	CELERY	41
ALMONDS	234	COTTAGE CHEESE	94	CASHEWS	38
BREWER'S YEAST	210	SALMON, CANNED	87	RYE GRAIN, BARLEY	38
SPRING GREENS	210	SOYBEANS, COOKED	73	CARROT	37
WATERCRESS	220	PECANS	73	SWEET POTATO	32
PARSLEY	203	WHEAT GERM	72	BROWN RICE	32
YOGURT, PLAIN	200	MISO PASTE	68	FISH	22

Calcium interacts with many other nutrients in addition to magnesium, especially vitamin D, and vitamin K, which aid its absorption and assimilation. We have already seen that high levels of magnesium will depress calcium levels; zinc, dietary fiber, and oxalates also negatively affect calcium absorption. Caffeine, alcohol, phosphates (very high in soft drinks and meat), protein, sodium, and sugar all increase calcium excretion and consequently reduce its levels in the body. Aluminum-containing antacids ultimately lead to an increase in bone breakdown and calcium excretion. Using aluminum cookware and aluminum foil (especially in the case of acidic foods) may similarly cause calcium loss. Calcium leaves the body mainly through renal (kidney) excretion, though losses also occur via feces, sweat, skin, hair, and nails. Apart from food, calcium also enters the digestive tract via the bile (from the liver), which is relatively rich in calcium, and in the pancreatic secretions. This is "endogenous" calcium produced from the breakdown of body cells, occurring naturally as cells die and are replaced.

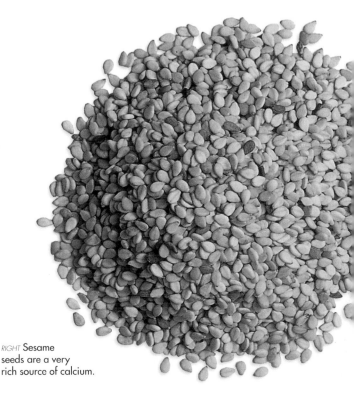

RIGHT Sesame seeds are a very rich source of calcium.

FUNCTIONS OF CALCIUM

- Essential for formation of bones and teeth (especially in pregnancy).

- Involved in nerve impulse transmission.

- Required for muscular contraction.

- Involved in the action of enzyme systems and cell communication

- Necessary for blood clotting and blood-pressure regulation.

- Essential for healthy heart function.

- Involved in the basic structure of cells.

- Has been used therapeutically to help menstrual cramps, cancer prevention, hypoglycemia, muscle cramps, osteoporosis, allergies, high blood pressure, migraine, heart problems, and insomnia.

DEFICIENCY SYMPTOMS

RICKETS IN CHILDREN	OSTEOMALACIA
TETANY	POOR TOOTH STRUCTURE
MUSCLE CRAMPS	IRREGULAR HEARTBEAT OR PALPITATIONS
LOSS OF MUSCLE TONE	HIGH BLOOD PRESSURE
OSTEOPOROSIS	COLON CANCER

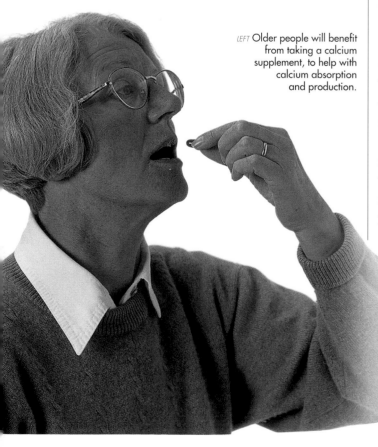

LEFT Older people will benefit from taking a calcium supplement, to help with calcium absorption and production.

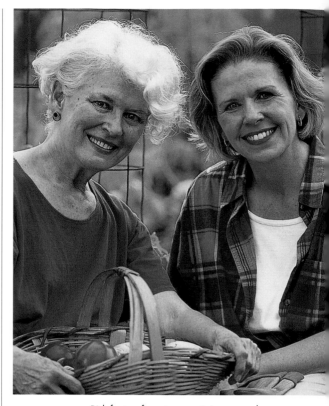

ABOVE Risk factors for osteoporosis increase where there is a family history of the disease.

CALCIUM SUPPLEMENTATION

Calcium is a "macromineral" and is therefore needed in very large amounts, the daily requirement being much greater than for other minerals. Because calcium is so important to so many vital biochemical body processes—blood clotting, muscular contraction, transmission of nervous impulses—it will be taken from our bones to satisfy these needs. This mechanism is under the control of parathyroid hormones. Removal of calcium from the bones and teeth can happen much faster in pregnancy when the growing fetus makes greater demands on the mother's calcium stores.

Obviously, bones will become thin and brittle as a result. In all those situations where demand is greater than intake, and if calcium taken from the bones is not replaced by calcium-rich foods or supplements, osteoporosis will eventually develop.

It is usual for the mineral calcium to be taken as part of a good quality multivitamin/multimineral complex, at a level of around 50 to 200mg per tablet/capsule. Extra calcium can actually be taken if symptoms dictate that it would be beneficial; levels ranging from around 50 to 500mg per tablet/capsule.

Calcium supplementation is used primarily in the treatment of osteoporosis, high blood pressure and muscle cramps. It may be supplemented in pregnancy to ensure adequate reserves for mother and baby. However, there are several other groups of people who are at risk of calcium deficiency and who would benefit from supplementation. These are the elderly (especially women), people on very low fat diets (impairment of calcium absorption), those using aluminum-containing antacids, highly stressed individuals (because of greater excretion rates), and women undergoing the menopause.

Calcium supplements are very variable both in chemical form and content. It is available as refined calcium carbonate, unrefined calcium carbonate (derived from limestone or oyster shells), calcium bound to various organic chelates (citrate, gluconate, lactate, amino acid), calcium orotate, dolomite, and bone meal. The absorption of calcium from calcium carbonate depends somewhat on the calcium becoming solubilized and ionized by stomach acid. This does not readily happen with calcium carbonate—the most widely used supplement, especially as stomach acid tends to decrease as we age. Also, some of the unrefined sources of carbonates have been found to be contaminated with other things, some of them potentially harmful like lead. The purest and most absorbable forms are likely to be citrate, amino acid chelates, or orotates. Doses over 2,000mg per day may cause hypercalcemia and some of this excess calcium may be deposited in soft tissues, blood vessels, and joints, if excretion is impaired. Since calcium works together with magnesium and phosphorus, and vitamin D is required for its uptake, these nutrients need to be plentiful in the diet or supplemented at the same time as calcium.

OSTEOPOROSIS

The major risk factors for osteoporosis in women are:
• Premature menopause.
• Postmenopause.
• White or Asian.
• Family history of osteoporosis.
• Low body weight.
• Short stature (and small bones).
• Low levels of exercise (especially in the late tee mid-twenties range).
• No pregnancies.
• Low stomach acid.
• Long-term corticosteroid therapy.
• Long-term anticonvulsant therapy.
• Hyperparathyroidism.
• Cigarette smoking.
• Heavy alcohol intake.

Osteoporosis occurs because of problems with both the mineral (calcium, magnesium) and the nonmineral (protein matrix) components of bone. It is much more than a disease related to lack of calcium alone. In adults, a low calcium intake resulting in calcium deficiency may, in fact, lead to bone softening—osteomalacia. In the disease osteoporosis, there is a decrease in the organic component of bone in addition to a lack of calcium, magnesium, and other minerals. Giving calcium supplements alone do not solve the problem.

Because bone is a living tissue, it is constantly being broken down and rebuilt as conditions dictate. Normal bone metabolism depends on many nutritional and hormonal factors, and the liver and kidney have a regulatory effect in addition to the overall control mechanism of the parathyroid glands, which keep blood calcium levels within very narrow limits. Estrogen and boron are also regulatory in preventing the excessive breakdown of bone tissue within our bodies.

There is some evidence that a vegetarian diet (both lacto-ovo and vegan) is associated with a lower risk of osteoporosis. Although bone mass in vegetarians does not differ greatly from meat-eaters in their 30s, 40s, and 50s, there appear to be significant differences in later years—decreased bone loss being the reason. Several factors may be responsible for this, the most probable of which is lowered protein intake. High protein diets are very acid-forming and this causes loss of calcium. Also, diets high in meat will be high in phosphorus, which also causes calcium loss. Refined sugars have been shown to increase the urinary loss of calcium, but, of course, such foods could be present in vegetarian as well as meat-eating diets. On the whole, vegetarian diets are likely to contain a greater amount of trace minerals, many of which will be involved in bone maintenance.

BELOW Choose foods like bean curd, nuts, and figs instead of cheese as a source of calcium.

MAGNESIUM

Quantitatively, magnesium is on a par with calcium and phosphorus in the body. Magnesium is likely to be far more important for a wider range of people than calcium, despite the media attention that calcium attracts. It is vital for many cellular functions, including energy production, protein formation and cellular replication.

ABOVE Cashew nuts also cont[ain] a good source

ABOVE **Peanuts** are rich in magnesium.

The primary function of magnesium is enzyme activation, but at least 60 percent of the body's magnesium is in the bones, where it is intimately involved with calcium and phosphorus in providing structure and strength. Muscle tissue contains about 26 percent of the total magnesium and the remainder is found in soft tissues and body fluids. The soft tissues with the highest magnesium levels are those that are metabolically the most active (brain, heart, liver and kidney) indicating this mineral's importance in energy production and synthesis of important biochemicals like nucleic acids and proteins. Muscle contraction requires both calcium and magnesium; calcium helps muscles contract, while magnesium helps them relax.

It participates in more than 300 enzymatic reactions in the body, many of which are involved in the production of ATP (adenosine triphosphate) the cellular energy store. Magnesium is required for the activation of tiny pumping mechanisms present in cell membranes; these help pump sodium out and potassium into cells. As a result of reduced magnesium levels, intracellular potassium is depleted and cellular metabolism is very greatly disrupted. Magnesium plays a part in blocking the entry of calcium into heart muscle and involuntary muscle cells lining blood vessels. In so doing, it can prevent vascular constriction and spasm which in turn lowers resistance to blood flow, reduces blood pressure, and improves heart function. Magnesium also helps regulate calcium metabolism via its actions on the parathyroid hormone and calcitonin.

MAGNESIUM CONTENT IN FOOD

The best dietary sources of magnesium are whole grains, nuts, seeds, and bean curd. Green leafy vegetables also provide good levels of magnesium, whereas fish, meat, and milk are quite low in this mineral. Western diets are likely to be very deficient in magnesium since meat, milk, and refined foods are commonly eaten. High consumption of tea and coffee can deplete magnesium levels even further. Women on the contraceptive pill and individuals suffering from chronic diarrhea, irritable bowel, and those using laxatives will also have compromised magnesium levels. Emotional stress and overexercising will add to magnesium loss and subsequent deficiency.

ABOVE **Magnesium and calcium occur in broccoli.**

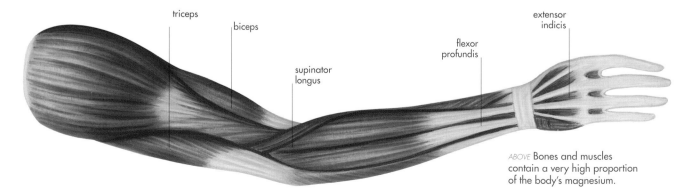

triceps

biceps

supinator longus

flexor profundis

extensor indicis

ABOVE **Bones and muscles contain a very high proportion of the body's magnesium.**

DIETARY REFERENCE VALUES FOR MAGNESIUM

	rni mg/day	rda mg/day
0–3 MONTHS	55	40
4–6 MONTHS	60	40
7–9 MONTHS	75	60
10–12 MONTHS	80	60
1–3 YEARS	85	80
4–6 YEARS	120	120
7–10 YEARS	200	170
11–14 YEARS	280	270 (males) 280 (females)
15–18 YEARS	300	400 (males) 300 (females)
19 + YEARS (MALES)	300	350
19 + YEARS (FEMALES)	270	280
PREGNANCY	270	320
LACTATION	320	280

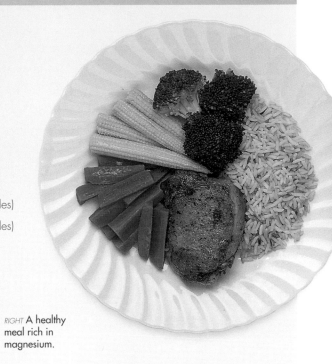

RIGHT A healthy meal rich in magnesium.

DIETARY SOURCES OF MAGNESIUM MG/100G

KELP	760	BROWN RICE	88	CAULIFLOWER	24
WHEAT BRAN	490	BREAD, WHOLE-WHEAT	76	CARROTS	23
WHEAT GERM	336	APRICOTS, DRIED	62	FISH, WHITE	23
ALMONDS	270	CORN	48	CELERY	22
CASHEWS	267	AVOCADO	45	CHICKEN	21
MOLASSES, BLACKSTRAP	258	PARSLEY	41	ASPARAGUS	20
BUCKWHEAT	229	SUNFLOWER SEEDS	38	BEEF, STEWING STEAK	18
BRAZIL NUTS	225	BARLEY	37	POTATOES	17
HAZELNUTS	184	DANDELION LEAVES	36	TOMATOES	14
PEANUTS, ROASTED	180	GARLIC	36	ORANGES	13
MILLET	162	GREEN PEAS, FRESH	35	MILK, WHOLE	13
PECANS	142	SWEET POTATO	31	EGGS	12
RYE	115	BLACKBERRIES	30		
BEAN CURD	111	BROCCOLI FLORETS	28		
COCONUT, DRIED	90	CHEESE, CHEDDAR	25		

FUNCTIONS OF MAGNESIUM

- Essential for bone structure and strength.

- Essential for cellular replication.

- Essential for production of energy.

- Necessary for hormonal activity.

- Balances and regulates calcium, potassium, and sodium.

- Helps bind calcium to tooth enamel.

- Helps to prevent diabetes.

- Required for muscular function.

- Required for heart function.

- Required for transmission of nerve impulses.

- Helps to prevent kidney stones and gallstones.

Used therapeutically to help in the treatment of:

- Asthma and chronic obstructive pulmonary disease.

- Cardiovascular disease.

- Acute myocardial infarction.

- Angina.

- Cardiac arrhythmias.

- Congestive heart failure.

- High blood pressure.

- Intermittent claudication.

- Low HDL cholesterol levels.

- Mitral valve prolapse.

- Stroke.

- Diabetes.

- Chronic fatigue syndrome.

- Fibromyalgia.

- Glaucoma.

- Hearing loss.

- Hypoglycemia.

- Kidney stones and gallstones.

- Migraine.

- Osteoporosis.

- Complications of pregnancy (including pre-eclampsia).

- Premenstrual syndrome and dysmenorrhea.

DEFICIENCY SYMPTOMS OF MAGNESIUM

Magnesium deficiency is extremely common in Britain and the United States, particularly in the geriatric population and in women during the premenstrual period. Low magnesium levels often go unnoticed because of reliance on serum magnesium levels to indicate status. However, most of the body's magnesium lies within cells, not in the serum, so that when low magnesium is detected in the serum, deficiency has reached a more severe stage.

Deficiency is often secondary to factors that reduce absorption (or increase excretion), such as high calcium intake, excessive alcohol consumption, surgery, digestive irritation, diuretic use, liver disease, kidney disease, and use of oral contraceptives. Low levels of magnesium both in the body and in the diet increase susceptibility to several diseases including heart disease, high blood pressure, kidney stones, chronic fatigue, cancer, insomnia, menstrual cramps, and PMS.

Pre-existing conditions that are associated with causing magnesium deficiency are:

- Pancreatitis.
- Congestive heart failure.
- Digitalis toxicity.
- Excessive sweating.
- Ileal resection.

DEFICIENCY SYMPTOMS

MUSCLE CRAMPS

MENSTRUAL CRAMPS

PMS

SUGAR CRAVINGS

FATIGUE

PALPITATIONS

NERVOUSNESS

DIFFICULTY RELAXING MUSCLES

ANOREXIA

ANEMIA

ANXIETY

FACIAL TICS

HYPOGLYCEMIA

HYPERACTIVITY (IN CHILDREN)

HIGH BLOOD PRESSURE

POOR CIRCULATION

KIDNEY STONES

LEFT Magnesium deficiency can cause excessive menstrual cramps and PMS.

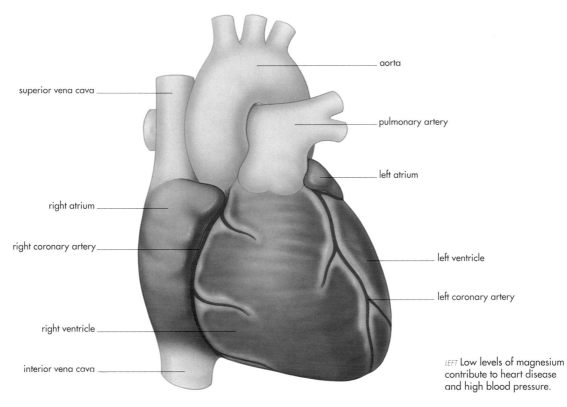

superior vena cava

right atrium

right coronary artery

right ventricle

interior vena cava

aorta

pulmonary artery

left atrium

left ventricle

left coronary artery

LEFT Low levels of magnesium contribute to heart disease and high blood pressure.

MAGNESIUM SUPPLEMENTATION

Magnesium, calcium, potassium, and other minerals interact extensively, so that levels of these will reduce the intake of magnesium and vice versa. In many enzyme systems where magnesium plays a role, vitamin B6 is needed to help increase the intracellular accumulation of magnesium. Because of these interactions, it would be safer to take magnesium as part of a multiformula, where levels might range from 50 to 100mg of magnesium per tablet/capsule. If symptoms are severe, an additional supplement of magnesium can be taken within the range of 50 to 300mg per day, but even this would be better in the form of a balanced mineral complex, to be used in conjunction with a broad spectrum multiformula. When single minerals are taken at high dosages, it can impair the absorption of other important minerals.

In general, magnesium supplements are well tolerated and absorbed—exceptions include magnesium sulfate (Epsom salts), magnesium hydroxide, magnesium oxide, magnesium carbonate, and magnesium chloride, all of which may cause diarrhea. Magnesium in the form of aspartate or ethanolamine phosphate are good highly absorbable complexes; or any of the Kreb's cycle (energy production cycle) intermediaries bound to magnesium such as citrate, fumarate, malate, succinate.

Drugs affecting magnesium levels include many diuretics, insulin, and digitalis.

Individuals with kidney disease or severe heart disease should not take magnesium supplements unless under the supervision of a physician.

CLINICAL REPORT

Numerous studies have shown that there is an inverse correlation between water hardness and high blood pressure—in hard water areas where water content of magnesium is high, there are fewer cases of high blood pressure and heart disease. More extensive dietary research has confirmed this effect. One of the most extensive studies in Honolulu found that there was around a 6.4mm of mercury systolic and 3.1mm of mercury diastolic blood pressure difference between the lowest magnesium intake group and the highest.

RIGHT High magnesium content in water may help prevent heart disease.

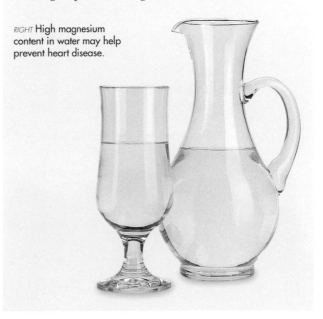

PHOSPHORUS

Phosphorus is essential for the structure and rigidity of bones. Combined with calcium, as calcium phosphate, the bone structure contains about 80 percent of the total body content, between 600 and 900g.

LEFT Whole grains, nuts, and soy products are rich sources of phosphorus.

The remaining phosphorus is found in the soft tissues as inorganic phosphate and as a constituent of all major classes of biochemical compounds, the most common being the energy substrate adenosine triphosphate (ATP), and the nucleic acids DNA and RNA, found in all body cells.

Phosphorus deficiency is extremely rare, despite it being required in fairly large amounts. Some chronic conditions can, however, lead to low levels in the body. Symptoms of such conditions are:

DEFICIENCY SYMPTOMS

DEBILITY	SPEECH PROBLEMS
MENTAL CONFUSION	ANEMIA
LOSS OF APPETITE	LOWERED RESISTANCE TO INFECTION
GENERALIZED WEAKNESS	
	OSTEOMALACIA

DIETARY REFERENCE VALUES FOR PHOSPHORUS

Phosphorus requirements are considered to be exactly the same as calcium, so that the ratio is 1:1. Therefore, the numerical values for phosphorus RNI and RDA are the same as that found in the table for calcium on page 80.

FUNCTIONS OF PHOSPHORUS

- Essential for the structure of bones and teeth.
- Essential for the structure of cell membranes.
- Essential for all major biochemicals in the body (and therefore energy production, cell replication, and all other metabolic reactions).
- Essential for communication between cells.
- Acts as a cofactor for many enzymes.
- Activates B-complex vitamins.
- Has been used as a special ergogenic aid for athletes.

DIETARY SOURCES OF PHOSPHORUS

As phosphate is a major constituent of all plant and animal cells, phosphorus is present in all natural foods. It is also found in great quantities in soft drinks, fast foods, and many food additives. Excess dietary phosphate will cause calcium depletion because of their antagonistic relationship. To prevent this, fast food sources should be kept to an absolute minimum. Natural foods containing a high level of phosphorus include meat, fish, whole grains, cheese, soy products, and nuts. The average daily intake in America is about 1,500mg for males and 1,000mg for females; in Britain it is very similar—1,200 to 1,300mg for adults. Since the adult RNI for phosphorus (and calcium) is around 700mg per day, the average Westerner has almost double the required intake and calcium depletion is certainly very likely.

Absorption of phosphorus is around 60 percent of intake and if dietary intake of phosphorus falls, urinary excretion is reduced, so that the body is able to regulate and maintain its phosphorus levels.

LEFT Cheese contains phosphorus.

COBALT

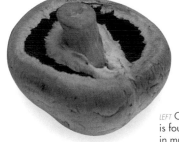

Cobalt is an essential trace mineral which forms part of the chemical structure of vitamin B12—cobalamin. It is in this "organic" form that cobalt is utilized. The functions of cobalt are, therefore, those of vitamin B12.

LEFT Cobalt is found in mushrooms.

Vitamin B12 is needed by the body to help maintain a healthy nervous system in addition to its roles in production of red blood cells and the utilization of fats, carbohydrates, and proteins.

DIETARY SOURCES OF COBALT

Good sources of cobalt are meat, liver, milk, oysters, and clams. Other foods high in cobalt will be those foods that are high in vitamin B12. However, some plants will carry cobalt in the soil particles that adhere to them. Vitamin B12 foods include almost all animal products, certain algae (edible seaweeds), and bacteria that can synthesize it from the cobalt in the soil. Land plants contain none at all unless they become contaminated by bacteria or algae, though some mushrooms like shiitake have moderate amounts. Therefore, vegetarians (and especially vegans) may be deficient in cobalt/B12 unless they consume large amounts of seaweeds, mushrooms, and fermented foods, or take vitamin B12 supplements.

FUNCTIONS OF COBALT

Forms part of vitamin B12. Used therapeutically as part of vitamin B12 to prevent pernicious anemia, to help in red cell production and for nervous system problems.

DEFICIENCY SYMPTOMS

There are no specific deficiency symptoms of cobalt; any deficiencies will be related to the activity of vitamin B12 (*see* page 50).

SUPPLEMENTATION OF COBALT

Cobalt is rarely found in supplements as a nutrient in its own right, except, perhaps, in multiformulas and those containing vitamin B12. When used therapeutically, side effects, such as goiter, hypothyroidism, nausea, kidney and nerve damage, and heart failure, occur at doses of 30mg and above.

DIETARY REFERENCE VALUES FOR COBALT

Since cobalt is part of the vitamin B12 molecule, requirements for this mineral are included as part of the vitamin B12 requirement—the RNI for an adult is 1.5mcg per day (see page 48).

LEFT Oysters, clams, and seaweed are a rich source of cobalt.

POTASSIUM

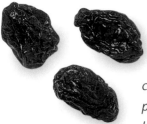

Potassium works with sodium and chloride as an electrolyte (a mineral salt that conducts electricity when dissolved in water). Electrolytes are crucial to the balance of body fluids and the control of the acid/alkaline levels. Additionally, potassium plays a vital role in the regulation and functioning of the heartbeat, protein synthesis, nucleic acid synthesis, conversion of blood sugar into glycogen, nerve conduction, energy production, and muscle contraction.

ABOVE Raisins have very high potassium but low sodium levels.

Potassium is predominantly an intracellular positive ion and is kept separate from, and in balance with, sodium, another positive ion, outside cells in the tissue fluid. Chloride ions, being negatively charged, balance sodium and potassium. Chloride is particularly important for the formation of stomach acid—hydrochloric acid. Potassium is easily lost in sweat and needs to be replenished after heavy exercise. The expensive "sports drink" manufacturers have fruitfully explored this aspect of sport physiology but a healthier, and cheaper, way to return the correct potassium/sodium balance is brought about by eating fresh fruit and drinking vegetable juices.

To maintain the compartmentalization of potassium and sodium, cells actually pump out the sodium that enters the cells and pump potassium into the cell. The pumping mechanism is found within the cell membranes and is called the "sodium–potassium pump." One of the pump's most important functions is to prevent cellular swelling. If sodium is not pumped out, water accumulates in the cell, causing it to swell and eventually burst.

RIGHT Bananas are a convenient and tasty source of potassium.

DIETARY REFERENCE VALUES FOR POTASSIUM

	rni mg/day
0–3 MONTHS	800
4–6 MONTHS	850
7–12 MONTHS	700
1–3 YEARS	800
4–6 YEARS	1,100
7–10 YEARS	2,000
11–14 YEARS	3,100
15+ YEARS	3,500

The safe and adequate intake set by the US RDA committee is 1,900mg to 5,600mg/day.

LEFT A salmon steak has a ratio of about 4:1 potassium to sodium.

Another function of the pumping mechanism is to maintain electrical charge across the cell membrane—this is particularly important in nerve and muscle function. It is not surprising, therefore, that potassium is vital for fluid balance and proper muscular contraction. A potassium

DIETARY SOURCES OF POTASSIUM IN COMPARISON TO SODIUM MG/100G		
	Potassium	Sodium
RAISINS	860	52
POTATOES	782	6
AVOCADO	680	5
LIMA BEANS, COOKED	581	1
SALMON	472	124
BANANA	440	1
COD	431	116
PORK	360	65
CAULIFLOWER	350	8
APRICOTS, DRIED	318	9
TOMATOES	290	3
CHICKEN	290	75
TUNA, CANNED (DRAINED SOLIDS)	281	47
BREAD, WHOLE-WHEAT	230	560
PEAS, FROZEN	190	3
ORANGES	180	2
MILK, WHOLE	140	50
EGGS	136	140
CHEESE, CHEDDAR	120	610

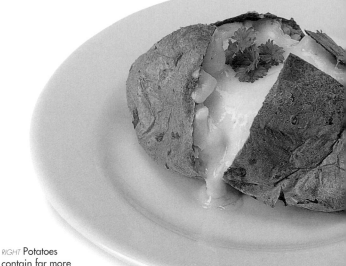

RIGHT **Potatoes** contain far more potassium than sodium.

shortage results in low levels of stored glycogen and, since exercising muscles use glycogen for energy, deficiency produces fatigue and muscle weakness. These two symptoms are the first two signs of potassium deficiency.

LEFT The avocados in a guacamole dip are rich in potassium and low in sodium.

POTASSIUM CONTENT IN FOOD

The total potassium content of food is important but, because of its intimate relationship with sodium, it is the balance of these minerals in food that has the greatest effect on physiology and health. Too much sodium in the diet will lead to a disruption in this balance. Much research has demonstrated that high sodium/low potassium diets are implicated in the development of heart disease, high blood pressure, strokes, and cancer.

The modern Western diet contains, on average, twice as much sodium as potassium. Moreover, this sodium is not the natural form found in fresh whole foods, but mostly comes from processing, cooking, and adding condiments to a prepared meal. When the levels are reversed, this degenerative disease pattern is prevented and, in the case of high blood pressure, a high potassium/low sodium diet acts therapeutically and reduces blood pressure considerably. Research shows that merely reducing sodium is not sufficient to cause this change—a high potassium intake must also occur. In fact, a ratio of 5:1 potassium to sodium is believed to be necessary for the maintenance of health and prevention of degenerative disease. Some experts say that this is still too low and that a diet rich in vegetables and fruits can produce a potassium-sodium ratio of over 100:1. For example, foods like lima beans have a 581:1 ratio, bananas 440:1, avocado 135:1, tomatoes 97:1, and potatoes 130:1.

As long as kidney function is normal, it is almost impossible to induce an excess of potassium by dietary intakes, although individuals with kidney problems may be advised to change their sodium/potassium ratios gradually over time. The amount of potassium lost in sweat is quite considerable, especially when exercising for long periods in warm environments. Athletes and those who exercise regularly have a high potassium, as do those people who live and work in a hot climate. Up to 3,000mg of potassium can be lost in a day through sweating; a daily intake in these cases needs to be at least 4,000mg.

FUNCTIONS OF POTASSIUM

- Necessary for correct fluid balance.

- Necessary for controlling acid/alkali balance.

- Required for protein, and nucleic acid synthesis.

- Required for the proper elimination of carbon dioxide.

- Essential for nerve and muscle function.

- Essential for heart function.

- Essential for adrenal and kidney function.

- Activates enzymes that control energy production.

- Prevents heart disease, high blood pressure, strokes, and cancer.

- May be of use in the treatment of cancer (Gerson Therapy).

- Has been used to help in the treatment of high blood pressure.

DEFICIENCY SYMPTOMS

WEAKNESS OF SKELETAL MUSCLES

HEART ARRHYTHMIAS

POOR PERISTALTIC ACTION OF THE GUT

MENTAL DEPRESSION

CONFUSION

POOR EXCRETORY FUNCTION (KIDNEYS)

FATIGUE

VOMITING

DIZZINESS

WATER RETENTION

EXCESSIVE THIRST

LOW BLOOD PRESSURE

DISTURBANCES IN NERVE CONDUCTION AND MUSCLE CONTRACTION

POTASSIUM SUPPLEMENTATION

Potassium supplementation is not normally recommended except as part of a full spectrum multivitamin /multimineral tablet or capsule. The reason for this is that by simply adding more of the high potassium foods to the diet, potassium levels can be increased considerably. Also, in an attempt to avoid extra sodium in table- and cooking salt, more potassium-based condiments are being sold and therefore used.

The two principal reasons for individual supplementation are for potassium depletion (when losses through urinary excretion, sweating, vomiting, or diarrhea exceed the rate of intake), and for helping treat high blood pressure. Severe potassium depletion can occur with the use of certain diuretics. Long-term use of some antibiotics (especially penicillin) may also deplete potassium and make a supplement advisable. In all cases where specific potassium supplementation is considered necessary, it should be taken, along with additional zinc and magnesium, only under the supervision of a practitioner. Otherwise, most people can handle high potassium intakes from the diet or multiformula since metabolism will quickly adjust to eliminate any excess. The exception is anyone with a history of kidney disease. These individuals process

BELOW To increase your potassium intake, simply add high potassium foods to your daily diet.

pyramids

ureter

pelvis

ABOVE Patients with kidney disease can have trouble processing potassium supplements.

potassium differently and may manifest heart disturbances and other symptoms of potassium toxicity. They should always discuss potassium supplementation beforehand with their practitioner.

Taking supplements to increase your potassium intake is contraindicated if you are already taking certain other medications, such as digitalis, potassium-sparing diuretics, and the angiotensin-converting enzyme (ACE) inhibitor type of drugs, which are used for lowering blood pressure.

CLINICAL REPORT

Many studies carried out have demonstrated that high blood pressure can successfully be lowered by increasing the intake of dietary potassium, which is readily available in a wide range of foods to satisfy those on meat-eating, vegetarian, or vegan diets.

One clinical study in particular cites a crossover study in which a group of patients was given either potassium or a placebo for a period of approximately two months before crossing over to receive the opposite treatment for a similar period of time. The results clearly indicated a significant reduction in both diastolic and systolic blood pressure in patients during the period of potassium supplementation.

Potassium supplementation may be especially useful in the treatment of high blood pressure in people aged 65 years and over. Some research (in a double-blind study) has shown that a four-week period of potassium supplementation (in a double-blind study) produces a significant reduction in blood pressure.

BORON

Boron is a "micromineral" or "trace" mineral since, unlike calcium, magnesium, phosphorus, or potassium, it is needed in very small amounts. It is a mineral that has only recently been recognized as being important for human nutrition. Preliminary results indicate that this nutrient may be helpful in maintaining healthy bones and joints. Recent evidence seems to indicate that boron is essential for the conversion of vitamin D to its active form. Additionally, it seems that boron reduces calcium loss by increasing the beneficial effects of estrogen and that this in turn improves bone health.

ABOVE Prunes are high in boron, but remain within the defined nontoxic level.

Boron is necessary for the activity of vitamin D—the vitamin that aids the absorption and utilization of calcium. Sunlight is also involved in the production of active vitamin D in the skin, and the liver and kidneys are further involved in biochemical changes to provide the most potent form—vitamin D3. Postmenopausal women with osteoporosis have high levels of the less active intermediaries, but low levels of the active D3, demonstrating an impairment in renal conversion.

Bones have been found to contain the highest concentrations of boron, but it has also been found in the thyroid and parathyroid glands. Its exact mechanism is not yet fully understood, although it is thought to play a part in improving bone density by its involvement in vitamin D3 production. Added to the diets of some postmenopausal women, it prevents calcium loss; this effect may be related to its ability to assist estrogen. Boron deprivation, after the menopause, leads to increased urinary excretion of calcium and magnesium and decreased levels of estrogen and testosterone in the blood. It is likely that boron is of great importance in preventing and perhaps treating osteoporosis.

BORON CONTENT IN FOOD

Fruits, nuts, pulses, and vegetables are the main dietary sources of boron. A diet rich in fruit and vegetables, in particular, is known to offer significant protection against osteoporosis. However, the level of boron in these foods will be totally dependent upon the levels of this mineral in the soil. Boron does not seem to be present at any measurable level in meat or meat products, but traces are present in dairy products.

Unfortunately, boron, like other trace minerals, is not a nutrient routinely added to chemical fertilizers, so that it is more than likely that overworked soils are

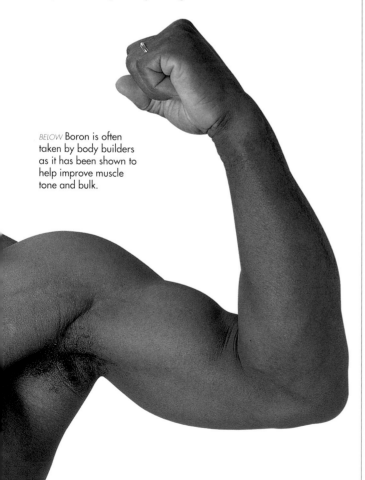

BELOW Boron is often taken by body builders as it has been shown to help improve muscle tone and bulk.

FUNCTIONS OF BORON

• Maintenance of bone density.

• Prevention of calcium loss in postmenopausal women.

• External treatment of bacterial and fungal infections (several natural antibiotics have been found to contain boron).

• Involved in muscle development.

• Associated with calcium, magnesium, and phosphorus metabolism.

• Used therapeutically to help to prevent and treat osteoporosis and arthritis, menopausal symptoms, and fungal and bacterial infections.

DEFICIENCY SYMPTOMS

SLOW GROWTH	POOR BONE MAINTENANCE
INCREASED EFFECTS OF STRESS	DEPRESSION

depleted; organic farming methods are likely to grow produce higher in boron because of their methods of fertilization. Cauliflower is a reasonable source of boron. In fact, it may be indicative of boron content in the soil since it grows very poorly in boron-deficient soil.

The level of boron intake in Americans is between 1.7mg and 7mg per day, but since there is not, as yet, any definitive intake recommended, it is not known if these levels are optimal. What is known is that the Western diet is particularly low in fresh fruits and vegetables—many individuals not reaching the recommended five portions a day—so that it is more than likely that some degree of boron deficiency exists in modern man.

BORON SUPPLEMENTATION

Based on available data, supplementation of boron may prevent bone loss. A United States Department of Agriculture study showed that supplementing the diet of postmenopausal women with 3mg of boron per day reduced urinary calcium excretion by around 40 percent and dramatically increased the levels of the most biologically active estrogen (17-beta-estradiol) a reliable agent for preventing loss of bone calcium. Some Australian research has also indicated reduction of symptoms of rheumatoid arthritis and faster healing of broken bones with boron supplementation.

DIETARY SOURCES OF BORON MG/100G

The figures for recommended daily intakes of boron are yet to be defined. So far, a level of up to 3.0mg has been indicated as nontoxic and safe.

SOYBEANS	2.8
PRUNES	2.7
RAISINS	2.5
ALMONDS	2.3
PEANUTS	1.8
HAZELNUTS	1.6
DATES	0.9
WINE	0.8

CLINICAL REPORT

Boron supplementation has been used in osteoarthritic treatment in Germany since the mid-1970s. In a double-blind study, patients were given 6mg of boron (as sodium tetraborate decahydrate) per day, and 71 percent showed an improvement compared to only 10 percent in the placebo group. From this and other studies, the indication is that boron supplements are valuable in arthritis and many people with osteoarthritis experience complete remission of symptoms.

The results of further research into boron's effects on osteoporosis are eagerly awaited.

There are several forms of boron available—sodium borate, boron chelates, or sodium tetraborate decahydrate. Levels can be from 3mg to 9mg of boron per capsule/tablet. Orally administered boron is extremely safe when taken at recommended levels (3–9mg per day).

BELOW An important ingredient in the Mediterranean diet, red wine contains boron.

CHROMIUM

RIGHT **Grape juice has a moderate chromium content.**

In 1957, an organic substance in pork was discovered which was able to restore glucose tolerance in rats; it was named "glucose tolerance factor" (GTF). Chromium was later identified as the active component in GTF, whose main function is to regulate the action of insulin, making it vital for the control of blood-sugar levels and thereby preventing fatigue and hunger. GTF does this by encouraging muscles and organs to take up glucose from the blood, when blood levels become too high.

Chromium is also able to stimulate protein synthesis and therefore increase muscle mass and bulk, boost resistance to infection, and control levels of cholesterol and fat within the blood.

Blood-sugar levels are balanced primarily by the pancreatic hormones insulin and glucagon. Chromium works closely with insulin in facilitating the uptake of glucose by the cells of the body. When chromium levels are low, GTF levels are low and the activity of insulin is blocked; blood glucose levels therefore remain elevated. Also, a diet high in carbohydrates will soon begin to exhaust the normal control mechanism. Imbalance will occur faster where stress levels are high because of the involvement of the adrenal glands. The end result is hypoglycemia, insulin resistance, obesity, and diabetes. Obesity is strongly linked to blood-sugar disturbances because of the decreasing sensitivity to insulin.

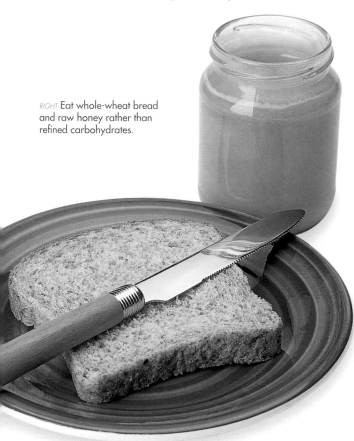

RIGHT **Eat whole-wheat bread and raw honey rather than refined carbohydrates.**

CHROMIUM CONTENT IN FOOD

Whole grains, eggs, and meat are the best sources of chromium. Fruits and vegetables have very low chromium levels. Since the body requires chromium, magnesium, and B vitamins to metabolize sugar properly, a diet that has excess sugar and other refined carbohydrates like white bread, white rice, and white pasta, will very quickly rob the body of these essential nutrients and create a number of deficiencies.

To prevent this, whole grains, high in chromium and other minerals, should be substituted for their much less healthy "white" varieties. Also, some research shows that lack of exercise can also deplete chromium levels, so increased activity might help with this. Chromium absorption is reduced by taking calcium carbonate or any of the antacid medications available.

FUNCTIONS OF CHROMIUM

• Essential for the regulation of blood-sugar, as GTF.

• Involved in maintaining healthy cholesterol levels; increases beneficial HDL cholesterol.

• Stimulates the synthesis of proteins.

• Helps increase lean muscle mass.

• Increases resistance to infection.

• Prevents arteriosclerosis.

• Used therapeutically to help in the treatment of elevated cholesterol and triglyceride levels, hypoglycemia, heart disease, diabetes, PMS, depression and anxiety, acne, and weight loss.

DIETARY REFERENCE VALUES FOR CHROMIUM

There are no definitive levels of RNI or RDA as yet. From various British studies and calculations, a range from 25 to 30mcg per day is considered to be the basic requirement for adults, while the American "safe and adequate range" is: children 20–120mcg/day, and adults 50–200mcg/day.

DIETARY SOURCES OF CHROMIUM MCG/100G	
EGG YOLK	183
MOLASSES	121
BREWER'S YEAST	117
BEEF	57
CHEESE	56
LIVER, CALF'S	55
GRAPE JUICE	47
BREAD, WHOLE-WHEAT	42
WHEAT BRAN	38
RAW SUGAR	35
RYE BREAD	30
HONEY	29
POTATOES, OLD	27
WHEAT GERM	23
GREEN BELL PEPPER	19
CHICKEN LEG	18
SPAGHETTI, WHOLE-WHEAT	15
APPLE	14
PARSNIPS	13
CORNMEAL	12
SPINACH	10
BANANAS	10
CARROTS	9
HADDOCK	7
BLUEBERRIES	5
GREEN BEANS	4

RIGHT Brewer's yeast is a rich source of chromium.

CLINICAL REPORT

Chromium can be an aid to weight loss. Some individuals who struggle with weight problems have become insensitive to their body's output of insulin. Since chromium can reverse this trend, it has been used by many in lowering body fat and increasing lean body mass. In one study, patients were given chromium picolinate at doses of either 200mcg/day or 400mcg/day, or a placebo. The study lasted around three months. The patients taking chromium picolinate lost an average of 4lb 3oz (1.9kg) of fat, whereas those in the control (placebo) group lost only 6oz (0.18kg). Furthermore, the group taking the supplement gained on average 1lb 6oz (0.64kg) of muscle as opposed to only 3oz (0.09kg) in the control group. The 400mcg dose did slightly better in these studies than the 200mcg dose.

DEFICIENCY SYMPTOMS

HYPOGLYCEMIA	HIGH BLOOD CHOLESTEROL
DIABETES (PARTICULARLY ADULT-ONSET)	ATHEROSCLEROSIS
FATIGUE	OBESITY
MOOD SWINGS	

CHROMIUM SUPPLEMENTATION

Many experts state that an intake of at least 200mcg/day of chromium is required. In some cases, especially therapeutic treatment of impaired glucose tolerance and obesity, 400 to 600mcg/day are routinely used. Diabetics should supplement with chromium only under their physician's supervision. There are several forms of chromium supplements available—chromium picolinate, chromium polynicotinate, chromium chloride and chromium-enriched yeast—supplying between 200 and 400mcg per tablet/capsule. All seem to work in a similar way. Chromium can also be taken as part of a multiformula. Toxic side effects of chromium supplementation are rare and since the absorption rate of chromium is usually low, there seems little chance that chromium supplementation would be unsafe. One study reported increased dream activity, greater vividness and color in dreams, and diminished sleep requirements with moderate chromium supplementation.

COPPER

Copper is the third most abundant essential trace mineral, after iron and zinc. The highest concentrations of copper are found in the brain and liver, but there are also appreciable amounts in skeletal muscle, the skeleton, skin, and bone marrow (where the blood cells are made). Bangles made of copper are often worn by arthritis sufferers, since copper appears to help the symptoms of inflammatory diseases.

ABOVE **Dried figs are a good source of dietary copper.**

Copper is an essential trace mineral that is involved in many key enzymatic reactions. It is a component of cytochrome oxidase and superoxide dismutase (SOD). These enzymes are respectively involved in energy release within cells and, along with all other antioxidant species, protection of cells from damaging free radicals. Synthesis of a range of neuroactive compounds (catecholamines and enkephalins, for example) also involves copper enzymes. Copper is part of the protein ceruloplasmin, found in the blood. This protein is active in regulating the blood level of certain hormones, in addition to helping in the formation of red blood cells. Copper is also involved in melanin formation to produce skin pigments, collagen production, and fatty acid oxidation.

COPPER CONTENT IN FOOD

Copper is widely distributed in a cross-section of nutritious food groups. In spite of this, however, most of our copper intake is not derived from food, but comes instead from copper-lined water pipes, cooking utensils, and from other potentially harmful sources such as processed foods, cigarette smoke, and pollutants (particularly from automobiles). Copper is also absorbed into the body by women who have been fitted with a contraceptive copper coil. In fact, in many cases copper intake exceeds the RNI, often being twice or even more than the recommended intake. Excessive copper levels have been linked to a range of disorders from schizophrenia and learning disabilities to premens-

RIGHT **A good reason to eat chocolate—it contains copper!**

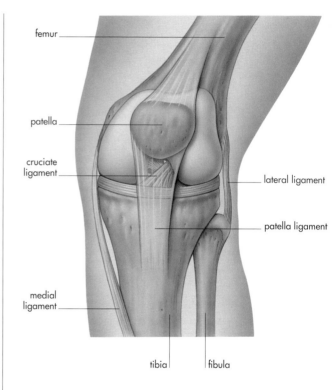

ABOVE Copper is essential in the production of collagen for healthy bones and cartilage.

DIETARY REFERENCE VALUES FOR COPPER	
	rni mg/day
0–12 MONTHS	0.3
1–3 YEARS	0.4
4–6 YEARS	0.6
7–10 YEARS	0.7
11–14 YEARS	0.8
15–16 YEARS	1.0
18+ YEARS	1.2
LACTATION	1.5

There is no official United States RDA for copper, but the safe and adequate range recommends: children (4–6 years): 1–1.5mg/day; adults: 1.5–3.0mg/day

DIETARY SOURCES OF COPPER MG/100G					
OYSTERS	7.6	SHRIMPS	0.8	OLIVE OIL	0.3
WHELKS	7.2	BUCKWHEAT	0.8	CARROTS	0.3
LAMB'S LIVER	6.0	PEANUTS	0.8	COCONUT	0.3
CRAB	4.8	SEMISWEET CHOCOLATE	0.7	GARLIC	0.3
BREWER'S YEAST	3.3	COD	0.6	BREAD, WHOLE-WHEAT	0.3
BRAZIL NUTS	2.3	TUNA, CANNED	0.6	PEAS	0.2
CASHEWS, DRY ROASTED	2.2	DRIED FIGS	0.6	MILLET	0.2
OLIVES	1.6	SUNFLOWER OIL	0.5	CORN OIL	0.2
HAZELNUTS	1.4	BUTTER	0.4	GINGER ROOT	0.2
ALMONDS	1.4	RYE GRAIN	0.4	MOLASSES	0.2
WALNUTS	1.3	BARLEY	0.4	TURNIPS	0.2
PECANS	1.3	PRUNES	0.4	PAPAYA	0.1
FIELD PEAS	1.2	MUSHROOMS, COOKED	0.4	APPLE	0.1

trual syndrome and anxiety. Fortunately, many of the potential problems inherent in copper can be offset by an adequate intake of zinc, since zinc and copper compete for absorption sites in the gut. Excess zinc decreases copper absorption and vice versa. Commonly, it is found that the foods high in copper are usually even higher in zinc (for example, oysters and other shellfish, nuts, and pulses) so that making these foods a regular part of the diet will help to maintain the correct balance between copper and zinc.

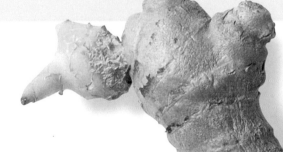

RIGHT Fresh and distinctive in taste, ginger root has a trace of copper.

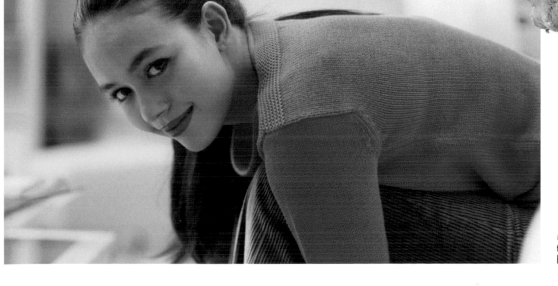

LEFT Copper should be taken by women who have a coil fitted.

FUNCTIONS OF COPPER

- A component of cytochrome oxidase; therefore involved in cellular energy production.

- A component of superoxide dismutase; therefore acts as an antioxidant against free radical damage.

- Involved in the synthesis of several neuroactive substances—for example, norepinephrine.

- Involved in regulation of certain hormone levels.

- Necessary for the production of adrenal hormones.

- Aids absorption of iron.

- Involved in the maintenance of blood vessels and nerve fibers.

- Essential for the utilization of vitamin C.

- Aids in tyrosine utilization for melanin production (for skin and hair pigment).

- Regulates cholesterol.

- Essential for red cell formation.

- Essential for the production of collagen; therefore responsible for health of bones, cartilage, and skin.

- Improves immune function.

- Inactivates histamine.

- Is used therapeutically to help in the treatment of cardiovascular disease and arthritis.

DEFICIENCY SYMPTOMS

ANEMIA	HEMORRHAGE
EDEMA	HIGH BLOOD CHOLESTEROL LEVELS
BRITTLE BONES	
IRRITABILITY	POOR IMMUNE FUNCTION
POOR SKIN AND LACK OF PIGMENTATION	

for the proper functioning of an enzyme needed for the crosslinking of collagen and elastin. Poor collagen integrity can also cause rupture of blood vessels.

Other signs of copper deficiency include brain disturbances, reduced immune function, increased lipid peroxidation, and elevated LDL cholesterol and reduced HDL cholesterol levels.

DEFICIENCY SYMPTOMS OF COPPER

Some of the features of copper deficiency in infants and young children include leucopenia, skeletal fragility, and increased susceptibility to respiratory tract and other infections. Anemia may develop if deficiency is prolonged and severe. Studies in adults suggest that some early features of copper deficiency can include defects in cardiovascular function.

Since several of the body's enzyme systems require copper as a cofactor, copper deficiency can affect several body tissues. It can produce iron deficiency anemia because copper is required for the absorption and utilization of iron. It can produce skeletal problems related to poor collagen integrity (for example, osteoporosis, and bone and joint abnormalities). The reason for this is that copper is needed

RIGHT **Crustaceans such as crabs and molluscs such as oysters contain high levels of copper.**

Copper deficiency may occur as a result of:
• Infant milk formulas low in copper.
• Intravenous feeding.
• Generalized malnutrition.
• High zinc intake (usually zinc supplementation).
• High vitamin C intake (usually from supplementation).
• Excess use of antacids.
• Chronic diarrhea.
• Celiac disease.
• Crohn's disease
• Increased loss (due to malabsorption problems, kidney disease, or burns)
• Chelation therapy.

COPPER SUPPLEMENTATION

Copper is available in many different supplemental forms, and it is up to the individual in question as to the form that they wish to take the copper in. It is also found in complexes with gluconate, sulfate, amino acids, and picolinate. All forms have been found to be of similar value. Copper is supplemented only when used therapeutically and under the supervision of a practitioner. Usually a diet high in whole grains, nuts, and fruit and including seafood and offal will prevent the need for supplementation, especially in those households where there are copper pipes.

Copper can also be found in multiformulas for general use, at a level of around 2mg or less. However, because of the common situation (at least in the West) of excess copper intake, many multiformulas can be found where copper has been deliberately omitted. Copper bracelets have been worn for arthritic conditions for many years now, since copper is absorbed through the skin. It has been found that the wearing of these bands can ease the aches and pains that are often associated with this debilitating disease.

Excess copper intake (as little as 10mg per day) can cause vomiting, diarrhea, muscular pain, and dementia. The lethal dose may be as low as 3.5g (3500mg), so it is very important that all copper supplements (as with iron) should be made totally inaccessible to children. However, chronic copper toxicity is rare, and a daily moderate intake is probably safe, but long-term supplementation may affect zinc status.

Supplements containing zinc should be taken at a different time of the day from copper supplements. However, if both are present in a multiformula, they generally occur in ideal amounts that will favorably enhance uptake and usage of both.

Large doses of vitamin C will also compromise the body's copper status.

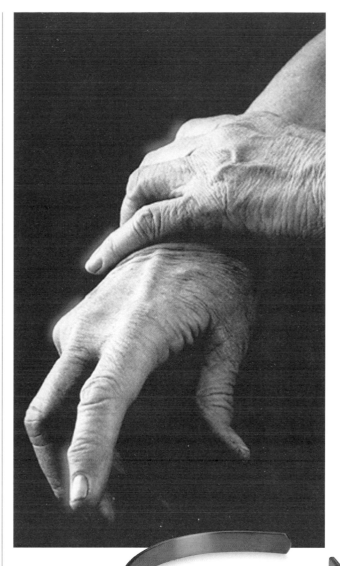

RIGHT AND ABOVE **Copper** bangles are worn to relieve arthritis.

CLINICAL REPORT

Copper deficiency, either because of low copper intake or excess zinc intake, may be a major risk factor in atherosclerosis. Elevated blood levels, damage to heart muscle, and arterial damage have also been related to copper deficiency. There is some evidence to be found in scientific literature to support these findings.

FLUORINE

Fluorine is a trace mineral found naturally, as fluoride, in soil, water, plants, and animals. It has been shown to be important in many body processes and may play a part in prevention of heart disease. Fluoride forms calcium fluorapatite in teeth and bones. It is involved in bone mineralization and assists in remineralization of bone in clinical demineralizing conditions. Its protective effect against dental caries seems to be intimately related to the presence of another mineral, molybdenum.

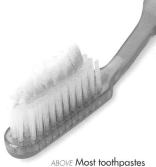

ABOVE Most toothpastes now contain fluoride to help protect against dental caries.

Excess fluoride can cause fluorosis, the most benign symptom of which is the mottling of the teeth with grayish patches. Some researchers have linked excess fluoride to overmineralization of the spine causing loss of flexibility, and even to cancer. Because of some of these worrying findings, the addition of fluoride to the water supply, which now occurs in many countries, continues to be an emotive and hotly debated issue.

DIETARY SOURCES OF FLUORIDE

Most foods contain very small quantities of fluoride, although some of these are trace. Particularly rich sources are seafood (including seaweeds) and black tea. In Britain, at least, the fluoride in food represents only about 25 percent of the total intake; the remainder coming from fluoride toothpastes.

ABOVE Mussels, like most other seafoods, are a good source of fluoride.

DIETARY REFERENCE VALUES FOR FLOURIDE

There is no RNI value for fluoride in the UK, but, because of its role in the prevention of dental caries, low-fluoride water supplies are flourized to a level of 1ppm (part per million), although many experts dispute that this is necessary and say that it may even be harmful. In Britain the mean intake in adults is 1.82mg per day from the diet, or 2.90mg per day if 1.1 liters of fluoridated water is included. High fluoride levels may be found in infant foods and, since children appear to retain more ingested fluoride than adults, an upper limit of intake for infants and young children is recommended of 0.05mg per kilogram of body weight per day. This is about 50 percent of the amount likely to cause fluorosis. The United States RDA is 1mg (3.6mg sodium fluoride)/day.

ABELOW Most foods contain traces of fluoride, but seaweed and black tea are particularly rich sources.

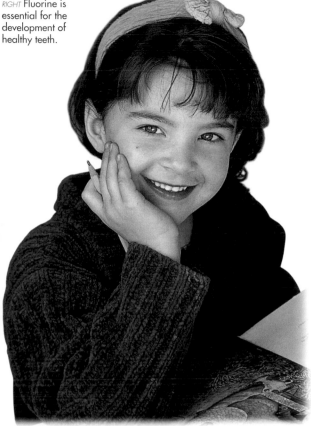

RIGHT Fluorine is essential for the development of healthy teeth.

FUNCTIONS OF FLUORIDE

- Essential for the formation of bones and teeth.
- May help prevent heart disease.

- Helps protect against dental caries.
- Protects against osteoporosis.
- May be helpful in the treatment of osteoporosis.

FLUORIDE SUPPLEMENTATION

Fluoride supplementation is not recommended without prior consultation with your physician or dentist. It is not usually found in multiformulas. If supplementation is deemed necessary, it should be taken with calcium.

In the United States, infants and children who received fluoride supplements of 0.5mg per day until three years of age and 1mg per day thereafter had a 63 percent incidence of fluorosis by the age of 12. It has also been found, in another study, that where the water supply naturally contains 1mg/kg, radiographic evidence of skeletal fluorosis has been reported in the adult population. Accidental exposure in adults to fluoride intake of 0.5 to 2.6g (500 to 2,600mg) per day over a short period of time gives rise to acute and potentially fatal fluorosis. Even doses as low as 10–80mg are considered toxic; serious tooth and bone problems and overstimulation of the parathyroid glands occur. Slightly lower doses than this range may cause energy and lethargy problems and lead to calcification of tendons and ligaments.

Tea provides 70 percent of the total dietary intake, so that those individuals consuming large volumes of tea are likely to have an intake of between 4.4 and 12.0mg of fluoride per day depending on whether or not the tea was made with fluoridated water. A study in the UK estimated, from information given in dietary records, that adolescents had an average intake (from water, soft drinks, and tea) of 0.96mg per day. Unlike most trace elements, there is a very small margin between beneficial and toxic levels of fluoride intake. Children who regularly consume too much fluoride may develop permanently mottled teeth. Chronic exposure to excessive fluoride may result in osteoporosis, calcification of the tendons and ligaments, and the growth of bone spurs, probably through the overstimulation of the parathyroid glands. Fluoride is also an inhibitor of the enzymes involved in glycolysis (cellular energy production). It may, therefore, have potentially adverse effects on energy production and its consumption should be particularly discouraged in those with chronic fatigue syndrome.

Fluoride in its ionic form is rapidly and completely absorbed passively from the stomach, but protein-bound organic fluoride is less bioavailable.

RIGHT Tea is a major source of fluoride in the diet, so heavy tea drinkers are likely to have a large daily intake of fluoride.

IODINE

Iodine is part of the thyroid hormone, thyroxine, which is produced by the thyroid gland and responsible for maintaining the metabolic rate. Iodine, which has a deep purple color, was first discovered in 1812 in the seaweed, kelp. It was extracted and named iodine, ion being the Greek word for "violet." It is also found in seafood and other seaweeds. Iodine deficiency is now rare in the UK, but it is still common in many areas of the world, including some parts of Europe.

ABOVE Plain yogurt is a quick and easy source of iodine.

Goiter (enlargement of the thyroid gland) affects over 200 million people throughout the world and is common in parts of the world where the soil lacks iodine. In such areas, iodine supplements or iodized sea salt is recommended to remove this problem. In the United States, the rate of goiter is around 6 percent in certain high-risk areas. Iodine is also needed for the integrity of connective tissue and modulation of the effect of estrogen on breast tissue. In the fetus, it is necessary for the development of the nervous system; infants born to severely deficient mothers are likely to suffer from cretinism.

IODINE SUPPLEMENTATION

Supplements occur as iodine or iodide; the body appears to handle these two forms differently. Iodides (sodium or potassium iodide) exert a stronger effect on thyroid function, whereas iodine is involved primarily in functions such as the modulation of estrogen on breast tissue. Natural sources of iodine are generally preferred to the iodides. Kelp supplements usually supply 150mcg of iodine per tablet/capsule. At doses of 750mcg, iodine has

been found to inhibit thyroid secretion, and people taking kelp to help weight loss should note this. Large doses may also aggravate or cause acne, and prevent formation of sperm. Iodine is toxic at very high doses. Generally, iodine is contraindicated for pregnant women, but may given under the supervision of a physician.

CLINICAL REPORT

Canadian research indicates that iodine (as iodine caseinate) may be effective in helping treat fibrocystic breast disease—mild to severe painful swellings in the breast tissue. Hypersensitivity to estrogen seems to occur in the absence of iodine, and this results in excess secretions distending breast tissue ducts. Small cysts form that later become fibrocystic. Treatment with iodine caseinate, at high levels, appears to correspond to a softening of the breast and disappearance of fibrous tissue plaques.

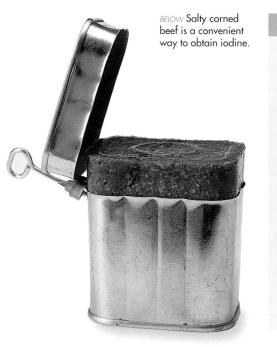

BELOW Salty corned beef is a convenient way to obtain iodine.

DIETARY REFERENCE VALUES FOR IODINE		
	rni mcg/day	rda mcg/day
0–3 MONTHS	50	
(0–6 MONTHS)		40
4–12 MONTHS	60	
(6–12 MONTHS)		50
1–3 YEARS	70	70
4–6 YEARS	100	90
7–10 YEARS	110	120
11–14 YEARS	130	150
15 + YEARS	140	150
PREGNANCY	140	175
LACTATION	140	200

DIETARY SOURCES OF IODINE

No accurate information can easily be given of the iodine content of plant foods because this is so highly dependent upon the soil in which they are grown. As a very rough guide, there is a maximum of around 10mcg/100g in vegetables and grains.

Other food sources are listed below:

DIETARY SOURCES OF IODINE (MCG/100G)	
IODIZED SALT	7,000
KELP, DRIED	5,350
HADDOCK, COOKED	200
MACKEREL	133
COD	100
PILCHARDS, CANNED IN TOMATO SAUCE	64
PLAIN YOGURT	60
HARD CHEESE	50
PLAICE, COOKED	33
SALAMI	15
CORNED BEEF, CANNED	14
ROAST CHICKEN	5

FUNCTIONS OF IODINE

• Essential for manufacture of thyroxine and triiodothyronine.

• May modulate the effect of estrogen on breast tissue.

• Helps relieve pain of fibrocystic breast disease.

• Involved in the integrity of connective tissue.

• Essential for proper development of the nervous system in the fetus.

• Can be used to protect against the toxic effects from radioactive materials.

DEFICIENCY SYMPTOMS	
SIMPLE GOITER	CHRONIC FATIGUE
HYPOTHYROIDISM	REDUCED IMMUNE FUNCTION
DRY SKIN	
EXCESS ESTROGEN PRODUCTION	

IODINE CONTENT IN FOODS

The use of iodized salt has reduced iodine deficiency in the UK and United States. Vegans not using iodized salt should ensure that seaweeds are regularly included in their diet; the Welsh delicacy, laver bread, is loaded with iodine. Iodine occurs in foods largely as inorganic iodides or iodates; these are very efficiently absorbed.

Storage and processing often cause a drastic loss of iodine. For example, a better way to cook fish is to bake, rather than boil or fry it. In Japan, where freshly caught fish is a dietary staple, iodine deficiency is almost unknown. In those areas of the United States and Europe where goiter still occurs, it is more probably owing to the ingestion of foods containing goiterogens, which block the utilization of iodine by the thyroid gland. Such foods include turnips, cabbage, kale, broccoli, mustard, cassava root, soybean, maize, bamboo shoots, sweet potato, peanuts, pine nuts, lima beans, and millet. Fortunately, cooking usually inactivates goitrogens. Manganese (from tea), and calcium, magnesium, and fluoride (in hard waters) are also considered to be goiterogens. Drinking large amounts of tea daily (five cups or more) will certainly affect iodine utilization.

DEFICIENCY OF IODINE

Severe deficiency of iodine in the expectant mother can lead to cretinism, intellectual disability, growth retardation in the fetus, also increased miscarriage, and increased infant mortality.

Iodine deficiency may be linked to Parkinson's disease, thyroid cancer, multiple sclerosis, and Alzheimer's disease.

ABOVE First discovered in kelp, iodine is also found in other seaweeds.

IRON

Iron is an essential trace mineral and is the second most abundant mineral in the earth's crust after aluminum. In human physiology, it forms the central part of the hemoglobin molecule within the red cells, where its function is to pick up oxygen at the lungs and transport it around the body to the tissues. It also transports carbon dioxide from the tissues to the lungs.

LEFT The spices that make up curry powder are very rich in iron.

A form of hemoglobin, called myoglobin, is found in the muscles. This is vital for immediate energy production in rapidly contracting muscles. Iron is an important cofactor in several key enzymatic reactions involved in energy production, general metabolism, and DNA synthesis. Iron-deficiency anemia is the most common mineral deficiency disease and was described by the Egyptians as long ago as 1500 BCE.

Because of menstruation and childbirth, iron loss for women is twice that for men. Heavy menstrual flow is associated more with a pre-existent low iron status than with it being the cause of the poor iron levels. Men can be iron-deficient, but for different reasons—peptic ulcers, hemorrhoids, or long-term use of antacids can all inhibit the proper absorption of iron.

Iron is stored in the liver, spleen, and bone marrow, ready for the production of new red blood cells. It has recently been cited as the mineral most lacking in those children with learning difficulties; presumably the reduced iron levels prevent appropriate oxygen distribution to the brain and other tissues.

BELOW Iron deficiency is implicated in learning difficulties in children.

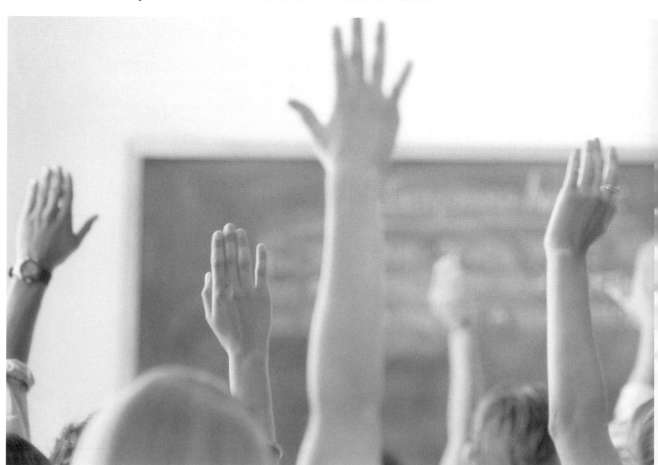

DIETARY SOURCES OF IRON MG/100G

KELP	100.0	SARDINES, CANNED	4.3	EGGS	2.0
CURRY POWDER	29.6	APRICOTS, DRIED	4.1	BEANCURD	1.9
COCKLES, COOKED	26.3	PRUNES	3.9	BEEF	1.9
BREWER'S YEAST	17.3	CASHEWS	3.8	WATERCRESS	1.9
FORTIFIED BREAKFAST CEREALS	16.7	TOMATO PASTE	3.5	KIDNEY BEANS, COOKED	1.9
MOLASSES, BLACKSTRAP	16.0	JERUSALEM ARTICHOKES, RAW	3.4	GREEN PEAS	1.8
PUMPKIN SEEDS	11.2	BRAZIL NUTS	3.4	DHAL, LENTIL	1.6
UNSWEETENED COCOA POWDER	10.5	BEET GREENS	3.3	BROWN RICE	1.6
WHEAT GERM	9.4	DANDELION LEAVES	3.1	OLIVES, RIPE	1.6
SOY FLOUR	8.0	WALNUTS, ENGLISH	3.1	BOSTON BAKED BEANS	1.5
LAMB'S LIVER	7.5	BREAD, WHOLE-WHEAT	2.7	MUNG BEAN SPROUTS	1.3
MUSSELS, COOKED	7.5	PILCHARDS, CANNED	2.7	BROCCOLI	1.1
SUNFLOWER SEEDS	7.1	GREAT NORTHERN BEANS	2.5	CAULIFLOWER	1.1
MILLET	6.8	CORNED BEEF	2.4	CABBAGE	0.6
PIG'S KIDNEY	6.4	CHOCOLATE, SEMISWEET	2.4	RED WINE	0.5
PARSLEY	6.2	SESAME SEEDS, HULLED	2.4	FISH, WHITE	0.5
CLAMS	6.1	LENTILS	2.1		
ALMONDS	4.7	PEANUTS	2.1		

DIETARY REFERENCE VALUES FOR IRON

	rni mg/day	rda mg/day
0–3 MONTHS	1.7	6
4–6 MONTHS	4.3	6
7–12 MONTHS	7.8	10
1–3 YEARS	6.9	10
4–6 YEARS	6.1	10
7–10 YEARS	8.7	10
11–18 YEARS (MALES)	11.3	12
11–50 YEARS (FEMALES)	14.8	15
19–50 YEARS (MALES)	8.7	10
50 + YEARS	8.7	10
PREGNANCY	14.8	30

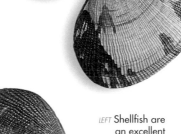

LEFT Shellfish are an excellent source of iron, and should be eaten regularly.

IRON CONTENT IN FOOD

There are two forms of dietary iron—heme and non-heme. Heme iron is bound to hemoglobin and myoglobin and is therefore found in animal products—liver, kidney, meat. Nonheme iron is found in plants, but it is poorly absorbed compared to the heme form.

Drinking coffee or tea within an hour of a meal can reduce iron absorption by up to 80 percent, but drinking high-vitamin C fruit juice with iron-containing foods will enhance absorption. Typical infant diets in developed countries (high in milk and cereals) are very low in iron. So too are the diets of adolescents consuming junk food.

Certain groups of the population are more vulnerable to iron deficiency: those with high physiological requirements—infants, toddlers, adolescents, pregnant women; those with high losses—menstruating women and those giving birth; those with poor absorption—the elderly; those with chronic diarrhea, malabsorption diseases, and low stomach acid; those who regularly use antacids; and those consuming inhibitor foods (such as tannin in tea). All of these groups, and possibly some vegetarians and vegans who consume the non-heme iron only, will need to consider improving iron intake.

Iron balance is regulated by both uptake and transfer across the intestinal lining. It is lost from the body in cells from the intestinal lining, bile, urine, and sweat, though losses via sweat, in comparison, are low. The amount lost will, however, be increased by those who exercise strenuously. Blood loss, by whatever means, obviously depletes the body of iron.

A diet typical for most non-vegetarians in industrialized countries comprises generous quantities of easily absorbed iron in the form of meat, poultry, fish, and/or foods containing high amounts of vitamin C to further

BELOW **For most us of us, poultry is the easiest way to get iron in our diet.**

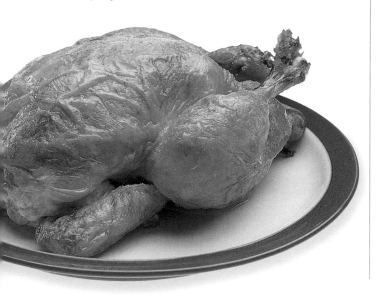

FACTORS AFFECTING IRON ABSORPTION

Inhibit Absorption	Increase Absorption
Tannins (in tea, etc.)	Vitamin C (ascorbic acid)
Polyphenols (in red wine, etc.)	Citric acid (in citrus fruit, etc.)
Phosphates (in soft drinks, etc.)	Lactic acid (in yogurt and milk)
Phytates (in cereals)	Malic acid (in fruit, etc.)
Wheat bran	Tartaric acid (in tart fruits and baking powders)
Lignin (in fibrous vegetables)	Fructose (fruit sugar)
Legume protein	Sorbitol (in diabetic foods, fruit, etc.)
Calcium	Alcohol
Manganese	Cysteine (amino acid)
Copper	Lysine (amino acid)
Cobalt	Histidine (amino acid)
Cadmium (in cigarette smoke)	

Additionally, iron uptake will be enhanced during pregnancy, fasting, or when in an iron-deficient state. Iron absorption will be inhibited when the stomach is low in acid (achlorhydria), if copper-deficient, and when iron is at a high level.

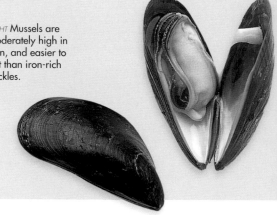

RIGHT **Mussels are moderately high in iron, and easier to eat than iron-rich cockles.**

FUNCTIONS OF IRON

- Essential for the formation of hemoglobin.

- Prevents certain types of anemia.

- Aids activity of many enzyme systems; especially involved in energy production.

- Necessary for immune function.

- Has antioxidant activity.

- Improves physical performance.

- Anticarcinogenic.

- May prevent learning difficulties in children.

- Is used therapeutically in the treatment of anemia, hearing loss, menstrual pain, restless leg syndrome, poor resistance to infection, fatigue, poor growth in children.

enhance absorption. However, iron in diets containing little or no meat is less well absorbed, even where the level of vitamin C is high. Obviously, then, many factors influence absorption and utilization of iron. If many inhibitors are present in the diet, the required intake of iron is raised; if enhancers are present, the intake of iron needed by the body will be much less. Also, although breastfed infants can absorb about 50 percent of the iron in milk, infants up to the age of three months fed on formula milks are thought to absorb only around 10 percent of the iron present.

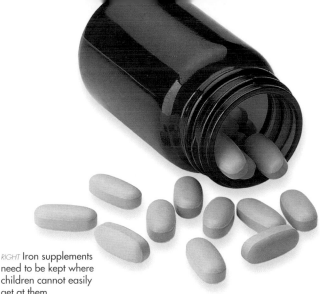

RIGHT Iron supplements need to be kept where children cannot easily get at them.

DEFICIENCY OF IRON

Iron deficiency ultimately results in defective erythropoeisis (red cell production) leading to anemia. However, functional consequences of iron deficiency may occur in the absence of anemia. These include: adverse effects on work capacity; poor intellectual performance; learning disabilities; behavioral problems; poor resistance to infection; and poor thermoregulation. These functional symptoms of deficiency are caused by poor delivery of oxygen to the tissues, a build-up of carbon dioxide, and the impaired activity of iron-containing enzymes in various tissues.

Iron deficiency is the most common nutrient deficiency in the United States. Infants under two years of age, teenage girls, pregnant women, and the elderly are at highest risk; 30 to 50 percent being iron deficient.

IRON SUPPLEMENTATION

Women of childbearing age are at the most risk of iron deficiency because of their monthly menstrual blood loss, but other groups may also need to supplement. Anti-inflammatory drugs such as aspirin and ibuprofen may also contribute to iron loss via gastrointestinal bleeding.

DEFICIENCY SYMPTOMS	
TIREDNESS	REDUCED BONE DENSITY
PALLOR	RESTLESS LEG SYNDROME
BREATHLESSNESS	POOR THERMOREGULATION
INSOMNIA	
PALPITATIONS	POOR RESISTANCE TO INFECTION
ANEMIA	REDUCED INTELLECTUAL CAPACITY
POOR GROWTH, BEHAVIORAL PROBLEMS, LEARNING DIFFICULTIES— IN CHILDREN	REDUCED WORK CAPACITY
SOME FORMS OF DEAFNESS	

CLINICAL REPORT

Several studies have clearly indicated that even mild iron-deficiency anemia can lead to a reduction in physical work capacity. Nutrition surveys in the United States have shown that iron deficiency is a major impairment of health and work capacity. Supplementation of iron demonstrated rapid improvements in performance.

Iron in the form of heme (organic iron) is the most efficiently absorbed (up to 35 percent). The absorption rate of nonheme iron supplements like ferrous sulfate and ferrous fumarate is much lower (around 3 percent on an empty stomach or 1 percent with food), and usually carries side effects like nausea, flatulence, and diarrhea. Nonheme supplements are also more likely to generate free radicals. Despite the positive reasons for giving the heme form, nonheme iron is still the most popular and tends to be the type prescribed by physicians. One of the reasons may be the lower absorption rate, since this will prevent overdosing and toxicity. The best nonheme form is ferrous succinate.

Iron can be taken as part of a multiformula at levels of between 1 and 15mg per tablet. However, since iron is often antagonistic to the absorption of other minerals (zinc, calcium, and magnesium), a separate supplement may be needed, though iron does need copper, cobalt, manganese, and vitamin C for its absorption and utilization.

Multiformulas without iron are available, if required, so that a separate iron supplement (supplying 15mg iron) can be taken at a different time. Children should take multiformulas only, not isolated iron supplements, unless under medical supervision. Iron taken as ferric iron will destroy vitamin E activity.

Toxicity is rare, but nonhem iron in excess can cause constipation. Children are at greater risk of iron poisoning so supplements must be locked safely away.

GERMANIUM

Germanium is not an essential mineral, and so far there is no sound evidence that it is essential to human life. But, "not essential" does not equate with "not useful." Several studies have indicated that many health conditions respond favorably to therapeutic doses of germanium—poor immune function, heart disease, arthritis, osteoporosis, and even cancer. Health professionals have used it in the treatment of Parkinson's disease, epilepsy, gastritis, arterial disorders, and as an anti-aging nutrient. Furthermore, the best organic sources of germanium are those very plants which are used by man for their curative powers; for example, ginseng, comfrey, garlic, and mushrooms.

ABOVE Garlic is useful for the treatment of many ailments.

Germanium seems to function by boosting the action of oxygen in energy production. A further development of this is the ability of germanium to maintain energy equilibrium; in so doing, it appears to reduce high blood pressure, lower cholesterol levels, and enhance the functioning of the immune system, thus improving resistance to illness. In this latter role it is behaving as a free-radical scavenger, or antioxidant.

Research by a Japanese scientist into the properties of germanium began in the 1950s. It was discovered that germanium was abundant in nature and that its richest source was coal. Since coal is produced from the compressed bodies of living organisms, including trees, germanium was considered to be an important life-enhancing nutrient. More research has revealed that germanium performs a variety of roles in plant life, such as: protection from viruses, bacteria, and molds; strengthening resistance to a cold climate; accelerating growth; and assisting in photosynthesis.

In humans, germanium appears to increase a balanced oxygen supply to the blood, thereby enhancing the body's resistance to viruses, such as that causing influenza, as well as mitigating the effects of auto-immune disorders, such as arthritis and rheumatism. Germanium was also found to stimulate the production of interferon. This is the body's natural virus-resisting substance and germanium is, therefore, seen to be of use in the treatment of viral illnesses. In addition, germanium appears to be an extremely effective painkiller, acting to prevent the breakdown of the body's natural opiates and prolonging their effect.

Many therapists believe that most health problems are related to a lack of oxygen; or rather an inability to regulate oxygen within the body. Germanium is unique in its oxygen-regulating capability and for the prevention of pro-oxidative reactions.

BELOW Eating foods rich in germanium can help the immune system fight off viruses much more efficiently.

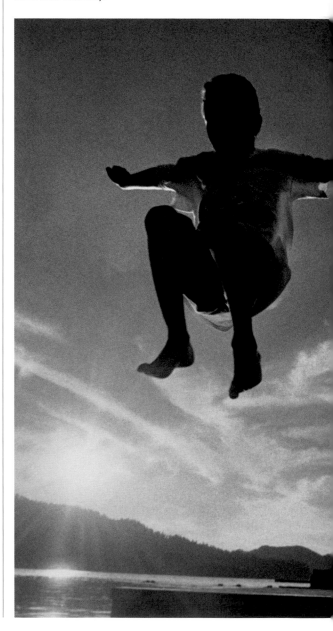

SUPPLEMENTATION WITH GERMANIUM

As a result of germanium's reported effects on immune stimulation, it was considered for use with AIDS patients and was available for a short time in the late 1980s as a dietary supplement in two forms: germanium sesquioxide (also known as organic germanium) and germanium lactate citrate. A third form, germanium dioxide, was not sold to the public as a dietary supplement because of its toxicity. However, some individuals in Japan did consume the dioxide form and suffered permanent kidney damage. The result was widespread withdrawal of all germanium supplements. Experts confirm that it may be virtually impossible to manufacture a completely safe, uncontaminated product. Therefore, the only way to obtain germanium is through diet.

Some evidence shows that germanium at doses between 50 and 250mg/day over periods of 4–18 months can cause serious harm and even death. There are no data to enable definition of a safe maximum intake.

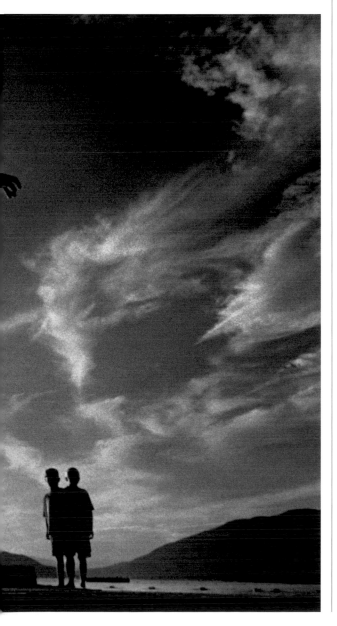

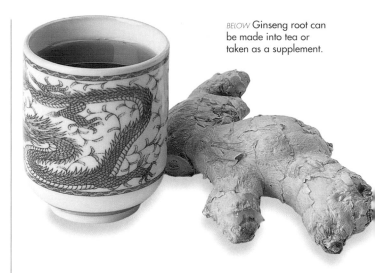

BELOW Ginseng root can be made into tea or taken as a supplement.

FUNCTIONS OF GERMANIUM

- Maintains a balanced supply of oxygen within the body.

- Acts as a powerful antioxidant.

- Protects against osteoporosis.

- A powerful immune enhancer.

- Protects against cancer.

- Natural analgesic.

- Anti-aging.

- Has antiviral, antibacterial, and antitumor activity.

- May help in the treatment of arthritis, candidiasis, influenza, bacterial infections (particularly of the gut), gut parasites, osteoporosis, Parkinson's disease, epilepsy, gastritis, and cardiovascular disease.

DIETARY SOURCES OF GERMANIUM

Germanium is an abundant element naturally present in the diet at trace levels of about 1mg/day. At this relatively low level it is excreted properly by the human body and is not harmful in any way.

Many often-used medicinal herbs are very rich sources of germanium—comfrey and ginseng are the best examples. The best food sources of germanium are garlic and mushrooms, particularly shiitake mushrooms.

ABOVE One of the best organic sources of germanium is mushrooms.

DIETARY REFERENCE VALUES FOR GERMANIUM

There are no official figures since germanium is not considered an essential nutrient.

MOLYBDENUM

Molybdenum is as essential trace mineral necessary for the functioning of the enzyme xanthine oxidase. This enzyme is involved in the metabolism and utilization of iron and in the production of uric acid (for excretion in the urine) from the breakdown of amino acids. Most of our molybdenum is stored in the liver, where the majority of its enzyme reactions take place.

ABOVE Lentils are an excellent source of this trace mineral.

Molybdenum is a component in several other enzyme systems, including those involved in DNA metabolism, alcohol detoxification, and sulfur metabolism. It also has a role to play in normal male sexual functioning, appears to have antioxidant activity, and is involved in excretion of excess copper from the body, since it competes with copper for its absorption

The body contains approximately 9g of molybdenum, most of which is concentrated in the liver, adrenal glands, bone, and skin. As with many minerals, increasingly sophisticated food-processing techniques and the destruction of the soil's natural vitality by pollution, pesticides, and unbalanced fertilizers, has drastically reduced molybdenum levels in our food and means that deficiency is today quite prevalent.

Low molybdenum levels may lead to increased allergic reactions to sulfites, commonly used in food preservation; many people are sensitive to this group of chemicals. The average person consumes around 2–3mg of sulfites daily in food, while wine and beer drinkers typically consume up to 10mg per day.

Several studies show that in areas where the molybdenum intake is high, there is a low rate of tooth decay. It has been found that the combined administration of molybdenum and fluoride is more effective in reducing dental cavities than water with added fluoride only.

MOLYBDENUM CONTENT IN FOOD

The dietary intake of molybdenum is between 50 and 500mcg per day. Pulses and whole grains are the richest source. However, the amount of molybdenum depends upon the soil content in which the plants are grown.

The rate of molybdenum absorption from the intestinal tract is between 88 and 93 percent, when dietary

DIETARY REFERENCE VALUES FOR MOLYBDENUM

There are no set RNIs, but safe intakes are considered to be between 50 and 400mcg per day for adults. The intake for breastfed infants of around 0.5–1.5mcg per kilogram body weight per day seems appropriate; children and adolescents (up to 18 years of age) should stay with this level.

In the UK, an average dietary intake for adults is around 128mcg/day; 48–96mcg/day in New Zealand; in the United States 44–460mcg/day (safe and adequate intake is 75–250mcg/day for 11+ years)

FUNCTIONS OF MOLYBDENUM

- Essential cofactor in many enzyme systems.
- Essential for metabolism of iron, sulfate, DNA, amino acids, and fats.
- Antagonistic to copper and enables excretion of high levels.
- Antioxidant activity.
- Involved in male sexual function; helps protect against impotency.
- Protects against cancer.
- Protects against dental caries.
- Reduces sulfite sensitivity.
- Prevents anemia; involved in iron utilization.
- Necessary for the amino acid taurine.
- Involved in detoxification of alcohol.
- Treatment of Wilson's disease (genetic disorder; increased storage of copper).

intakes are between 20 and 1,500mcg/day. At low dietary intakes, it is conserved by the body; when intakes are excessive it is usually rapidly excreted in the urine, so that toxicity through diet should not normally occur. There is some evidence that high dietary molybdenum intake of 10–15mg (10,000 to 15,000mcg) per day is associated with altered metabolism of nucleotides, symptoms of gout, and with impaired copper availability.

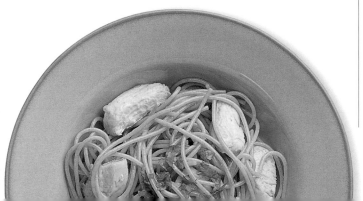

LEFT A dish of chicken and noodles will satisfy the daily molybdenum requirement.

DIETARY SOURCES OF MOLYBDENUM mcg/100g

BEANS, CANNED	350	BROWN RICE	75	BREAD, WHOLE-WHEAT	32
LIVER	200	GARLIC	70	POTATOES	30
LENTILS	155	GREEN BEANS	66	ONION	25
FIELD PEAS	130	OATS	60	PEANUTS	25
CAULIFLOWER	120	MACARONI	51	COCONUT	25
SUNFLOWER SEEDS	103	EGGS	50	SHELLFISH	20
GREEN PEAS	110	RYE BREAD	50	APRICOTS	14
BREWER'S YEAST	109	CORN	45	STRAWBERRIES	7
WHEAT GERM	100	NOODLES	45	CARROTS	5
SPINACH	100	BARLEY	42	CABBAGE	5
KIDNEY	75	CHICKEN	40		

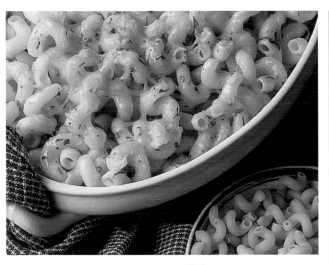

ABOVE Macaroni, made from semolina, contains molybdenum.

MOLYBDENUM SUPPLEMENTATION

Molybdenum supplementation has several possible applications, including sulfite sensitivity, cancer prevention, prevention of dental caries, and treatment for Wilson's disease. The dosage ranges for therapeutic treatment is 200 to 500mcg per day (strictly under a practitioner's supervision). Molybdenum is available as sodium molybdate; elemental molybdenum dose is suggested to be between 50 and 100mcg per day as a preventative nutrient. It is usually supplemented as part of a multiformula. A high intake of copper or ferrous sulfate can decrease absorption of molybdenum. Molybdenum is synergistic to fluoride and is relatively nontoxic at normal intake levels, but excess may cause goutlike symptoms.

CLINICAL REPORT

Some experimental findings have implicated molybdenum deficiency as a factor in some forms of cancer. One particular study carried out in China demonstrated that where soil molybdenum levels are low, the rate of esophageal cancer is higher. In the United States, there is a 30 percent increase in esophageal cancer in areas where there is no molybdenum in the drinking water. Studies on animals confirm that addition of molybdenum to drinking water can inhibit chemically induced esophageal cancer. The anticancer effects of molybdenum probably relate to its role in detoxification of carcinogens.

ABOVE Molybdenum is often added to mineral water with fluoride.

DEFICIENCY SYMPTOMS

INCREASED SULFITE SENSITIVITY	IRRITABILITY
IRREGULAR HEARTBEAT	INABILITY TO PRODUCE URIC ACID

MANGANESE

Manganese is an essential trace mineral and is involved as a component or activator of several enzyme systems, such as blood-sugar balance, energy production, protein and carbohydrate metabolism, and thyroid function. It is essential for the functioning of superoxide dismutase (SOD), which prevents the damaging effects of the superoxide free radical from destroying cellular structures and causing inflammation. Manganese is also involved in bone formation, muscular contraction, fertility, brain function, and inner ear balance.

ABOVE In the UK, half the daily manganese intake comes from tea.

MANGANESE CONTENT IN FOOD

Tea is estimated to supply half the amount of manganese in the British diet (around 2.4mg/day). Otherwise, whole grains, nuts, and avocados are rich sources, with fruits and vegetables containing moderate amounts. The milling of grains removes approximately 70 percent of the manganese. Meats, dairy products, poultry, and seafood are considered poor sources of manganese.

Absorption of manganese occurs throughout the whole length of the small intestine, but the efficiency of this process is low. High intakes of calcium, copper, iron, magnesium, zinc, and phytates in cereal bran may inhibit the absorption of manganese. Regular antacid use may also inhibit the absorption of manganese. Conversely, manganese is an inhibitor in the absorption of copper, iron, and zinc.

FUNCTIONS OF MANGANESE

- Essential for the working of many enzyme systems.

- Essential for glucose metabolism.

- Involved in protein metabolism.

- Important antioxidant.

- Involved in muscular contraction.

- Involved in brain function.

- Necessary for healthy bone and cartilage structure.

- Involved in the formation of thyroid hormones.

- Involved in fertility.

- Required to produce melanin.

- Involved in the synthesis of fatty acids.

- Helps in detoxification and the production of urea.

- Needed for proper balance (inner ear).

- May prevent osteoporosis.

- Used therapeutically to help in the treatment of strains, sprains, inflammation, epilepsy, diabetes, Alzheimer's disease, schizophrenia, myasthenia gravis, anemia, heart disease, atherosclerosis, and arthritis.

DEFICIENCY SYMPTOMS

Manganese deficiency leads to abnormal bone and cartilage growth, as well as a degeneration of the vertebral disks and might, therefore, play a part in the prevention of degenerative bone diseases such as osteoporosis. In studies, where volunteers were fed a manganese-deficient diet, symptoms of skin rash, loss of hair color, change of bone shape, reduced growth of hair and nails, and a reduction in the good cholesterol (HDL) occurred.

SUPPLEMENTATION WITH MANGANESE

Manganese is one of the least toxic of all the elements. When intake is excessive, it is excreted readily via the liver and kidneys. However, manganese toxicity from environmental pollution can become a serious health problem. In its most severe form, it produces severe psychiatric symptoms such as hallucinations, violent acts, and hyper-irritability.

As a supplement, it is available in various forms. Inorganic manganese salts such as manganese sulfate or manganese chloride do not seem to be as well absorbed as manganese picolinate, gluconate, or other chelates. The principal uses of manganese are: the treat-

LEFT A seasonal favorite, chestnuts are a good source of manganese.

DIETARY SOURCES OF MANGANESE MG/100G

WHEAT GERM, TOASTED	19.9	COCONUT	1.3	RAISINS	0.5
AVOCADOS	4.2	RYE	1.3	TURNIP GREENS	0.5
CHESTNUTS	3.7	BUCKWHEAT	1.3	RHUBARB	0.5
PECANS	3.5	FIELD PEAS, DRY	1.3	BEET GREENS	0.4
HAZELNUTS	3.5	LENTILS	1.2	LAMB'S LIVER	0.4
BUCKWHEAT FLOUR	2.1	LOGANBERRIES	1.2	BRUSSELS SPROUTS	0.3
BRAZIL NUTS	2.8	PLUMS	1.0	BOSTON BAKED BEANS	0.3
ALMONDS	2.5	WALNUTS	0.8	OATMEAL	0.3
PEAS	2.0	SPINACH, FRESH	0.8	CORNMEAL	0.2
BARLEY	1.8	PEANUTS	0.7	MILLET	0.2
BROWN RICE	1.6	LETTUCE	0.7	CARROTS	0.2
TEA (1 CUP)	1.5	BANANAS	0.6	BROCCOLI	0.2
BLACKBERRIES, STEWED	1.5	BEET	0.6	WHOLE-WHEAT BREAD	0.1
PINEAPPLE, CANNED	1.5	OATS	0.6		

RIGHT Bananas contain trace elements of the mineral manganese, as well as high potassium levels.

DIETARY REFERENCE VALUES FOR MANGANESE

There is no official RNI for manganese, but suggested safe and adequate intakes lie between 2.5 and 5.0mg per day for adults.

DEFICIENCY SYMPTOMS

POOR BALANCE

POOR MEMORY

DERMATITIS

IMPAIRED CARBOHYDRATE METABOLISM

NERVOUS IRRITABILITY

FATIGUE

BLOOD-SUGAR IMBALANCES

POOR HAIR AND NAIL GROWTH

HEAVY MENSTRUAL BLEEDING

REDUCED SEIZURE THRESHOLD IN EPILEPTICS

FRAGILE BONES

JOINT DEGENERATION

ment of strains, sprains, and inflammation (15–30mg per day); epilepsy (15–30mg per day); diabetes (5–15mg per day). For the treatment of epilepsy and diabetes, supplements must be under the supervision of a physician.

Manganese can be used as a separate supplement at 15mg per day or less, but is more often found as part of a multiformula at a level of between 0.5 and 5mg.

CLINICAL REPORT

Manganese is a popular nutrient taken for strains, sprains, and inflammatory conditions, because of its involvement in the antioxidant enzyme system involving SOD. Although manganese studies with regard to these conditions are few, manganese is assumed to be effective because its supplementation is effective in raising the levels of SOD in the body. There is evidence that individuals with rheumatoid arthritis need an increased intake of manganese.

SELENIUM

RIGHT Brazil nuts are an excellent source of selenium.

Selenium is an essential trace mineral which is now considered to be one of the most important nutrients. The name selenium is derived from the moon goddess Selene and the mineral was first regarded as a poison. It is now one of the most talked-about nutrients. It is a powerful antioxidant protecting against many cancers and age-related degenerative conditions such as heart disease, arthritis, cataract formation, and premature aging.

Selenium is beneficial in the treatment and prevention of some immune-deficient conditions and may, therefore, have a role to play in the treatment of HIV and AIDS. Its main antioxidant activity is as part of the enzyme, glutathione peroxidase, which works alongside vitamin E in protecting intracellular structures against oxidative damage by free radicals. It is of particular importance in liver detoxification. Selenium is able to inhibit the harmful effects of heavy metals such as arsenic, cadmium, mercury and lead. It is a mineral which has become very depleted in soils worldwide, so that very few foods now contain appropriate amounts and, consequently, supplementation is often the only way to boost levels appropriately.

In addition to glutathione peroxidase, other seleno-proteins have been isolated from mammalian tissues and their activities investigated. Of particular interest to the nutritionist is the role of selenium in metabolism of thyroxine in the liver.

There is substantial evidence that selenium is essential for proper fetal growth and development. Selenium requirements seem to increase during pregnancy and low levels are associated with low birth weight. Low selenium levels in the newborn have been tentatively linked to sudden infant death syndrome (SIDS), which, like heart disease and cancer, has the highest occurrence in areas of the world where the selenium content of the soil and within the diet is at its lowest.

However, the body requires only a very small amount of selenium, as can be seen from the dietary reference values. Despite this, there are many individuals who are consuming an insufficient amount of this mineral. Furthermore, since the required intake is low, supplementation must be undertaken with care. Acute selenium toxicity from dietary intake alone is very rare. (*For symptoms of this, see p. 118.*)

BELOW Paella has all the ingredients for a healthy intake of selenium.

DIETARY REFERENCE VALUES FOR SELENIUM	rni mcg/day	rda mcg/day
0–3 MONTHS	10	10
4–6 MONTHS	13	10
7–12 MONTHS	10	15
1–3 YEARS	15	20
4–6 YEARS	20	20
7–10 YEARS	30	30
11–14 YEARS	45	40 (males) 45 (females)
15–18 YEARS (MALES)	70	50
19+ YEARS (MALES)	75	70
15–18 YEARS (FEMALES)	60	50
19 + YEARS (FEMALES)	60	55
PREGNANCY	60	65
LACTATION	75	75

DIETARY SOURCES OF SELENIUM MCG/100G	
MOLASSES, BLACKSTRAP	130
WHEAT GERM	111
BRAZIL NUTS	103
CASHEWS, DRY ROASTED	67
WHOLE-WHEAT BREAD	66
BARLEY	66
SHRIMP	59
OATS	56
CLAMS, RAW	55
OYSTERS	49
COD	43
LIVER	40
BROWN RICE	39
SHELLFISH	32
LAMB	30
TURNIPS	27
GARLIC	25
ORANGE JUICE	19
BEER	19
PORK	15
MUSHROOMS, COOKED	12
CHICKEN, COOKED AND SKINLESS	8
PULSES	5
ZUCCHINI, RAW	3
BOSTON BAKED BEANS	2
CARROTS, COOKED	2

RIGHT Include turnips and rutabagas in stews for a boost of selenium.

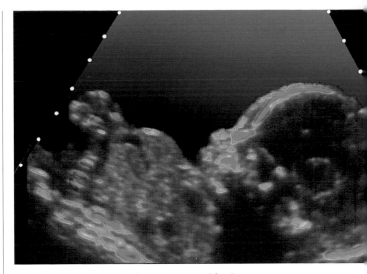

ABOVE Selenium is essential for the normal growth and development of the fetus in the womb.

SELENIUM CONTENT IN FOOD

Selenium is present in foods mainly as the amino acids selenomethionine and selenocysteine and their derivatives.

The level of selenium in plant foods is directly related to the level of selenium in the soil. Soils worldwide are becoming very depleted in this mineral. Especially deficient are soils found in the UK, Finland and other parts of Europe, New Zealand, and China. Cereals and flour from countries like Canada, where the soil is rich in selenium, are the best to buy if possible. Fish and shellfish are good sources of selenium, as are some meats, but again it depends on the selenium content of those animals further down the food chain as to the amount of selenium present in such foods.

Between 55 and 65 percent of selenium in the diet is absorbed from the digestive tract, and if intake is excessive —unlikely—unless supplementing—it will be excreted in the urine. The amount of selenium lost in urine, or detected in tissues and blood, is a direct reflection of dietary intakes. Thus, the selenium status of individuals correlates with the amount and availability of selenium in their diet and the soils from which they obtain their foods. There may be an increased requirement for those people who smoke, take the contraceptive pill, or have diets high in refined food. The elderly, adolescents, vegetarians, and pregnant and nursing mothers are those most at risk from low selenium intake, so that a frequent intake of foods like Brazil nuts, wheat germ, shellfish, and fish is needed. Selenium absorption is adversely affected by heavy metals (lead, mercury, cadmium) and high doses of vitamin C. There may also be some antagonism between selenium and other trace minerals like zinc. Various drugs, such as those used in chemotherapy, may increase the body's requirement for selenium.

FUNCTIONS OF SELENIUM

- Important antioxidant.

- Important for immune function.

- Necessary for DNA repair.

- Essential for healthy fetal growth.

- Involved in the detoxification of alcohol, some drugs, and pollutants, including smoke.

- Involved in male potency and libido.

- Improves liver function.

- Necessary for proper thyroid function.

- Protects against heart disease and circulatory problems.

- Maintains healthy eyes, skin, nails, and hair.

- Is used therapeutically to help in the treatment of dandruff, acne, psoriasis, cataracts, arthritis, asthma, poor sperm motility, thyroid function, kidney problems, muscular dystrophy, hepatitis, epilepsy, AIDS, cancers.

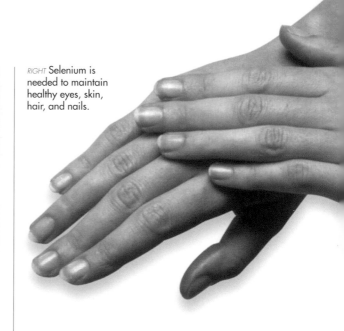

RIGHT Selenium is needed to maintain healthy eyes, skin, hair, and nails.

DEFICIENCY SYMPTOMS OF SELENIUM

Advanced selenium deficiency is associated with a severe heart disorder, called Keshan disease, which affects children and women of childbearing age. It occurs in areas of China where soil levels of selenium are very low and dietary intake is less than 12mcg per day. It is, however, very rare. More commonly, mild, chronic deficiency of selenium is associated with poor immune function, cardiovascular disease, and cancer.

SELENIUM SUPPLEMENTATION

Selenium is available in several different forms. Studies indicate that selenium in inorganic form, such as sodium selenite, is not absorbed as effectively as organic forms such as selenomethionine and selenium-rich yeast. Organic forms are also more biologically active. Selenium is available as a separate supplement in dosages from 50mcg to 200mcg per day.

More often, though, selenium is supplemented along with other antioxidant nutrients (with which it acts in the body; vitamins A, C, and E) at a dosage of around 200mcg per tablet. It is a common ingredient in most widely available multiformulas.

A recommended maximum safe intake of selenium from all sources (diet and supplements) is 450mcg per day for adult males. A safe maximum intake for adult females will be a little less than this. Levels of up to 1,000mcg per day have been used to stimulate immune function and prevent cancer, but this should be taken only under the supervision of a practitioner. There is some evidence that disturbed selenium balance occurs at intakes above 750mcg per day. Toxic signs have been observed in individuals taking 900mcg/day over prolonged periods. These symptoms include blackening finger nails, a garlic odor on skin and breath, depression, nervousness, emotional instability, and nausea and vomiting. In extreme cases, there can be loss of hair and nails. However, selenium toxicity from dietary sources is rare. The main uses for selenium supplementation relate to its activity as a powerful antioxidant, and include cancer prevention, immune stimulation, and protection against cardiovascular disease, inflammatory conditions, and cataract formation.

DEFICIENCY SYMPTOMS	
CATARACTS	REDUCED MALE FERTILITY
INCREASED SUSCEPTIBILITY TO INFECTION	MUSCLE INFLAMMATION
	AGE SPOTS
HEART PROBLEMS	HAIR LOSS
POOR GROWTH IN CHILDREN	POOR DETOXIFICATION

LEFT Barley and products made from barley are very rich in selenium.

CLINICAL REPORTS

IMMUNE FUNCTION

Glutathione peroxidase is an enzyme containing selenium. It is vital to immune function. The ability of selenium to enhance immune function goes further than just restoring the blood levels to normal. One piece of clinical research gave individuals, with normal blood concentrations, a supplement containing 200mcg/day. The results indicated over 100 percent increase in the ability of some types of white cell to kill tumor cells and microorganisms. Blood levels of selenium after supplementation were not significantly increased. These findings indicate that immune-enhancing effects of selenium require supplementation in addition to dietary intake.

CANCER

Researchers have found consistently low levels of selenium and glutathione peroxidase in the blood of patients suffering from many forms of cancer, compared to levels in healthy individuals. Some studies even produced data which demonstrated low selenium levels in people years before their cancers developed. The anticancer effects of selenium seem to be more significant in men than in women and are most important in the prevention of respiratory and gastrointestinal cancers.

HEART DISEASE

Rates of heart disease are highest where selenium intake is lowest. Selenium supplementation of around 100mcg/day appears to increase the ratio of good cholesterol (HDL) to the bad (LDL), and inhibits platelet aggregation. The protective action seems to be greater in smokers.

In one study, heart attack patients were randomly assigned either 100mcg selenium per day or a placebo. After six months, there were six times more heart attacks in the placebo group than there were in the selenium group.

RIGHT Selenium is required in the diet to ensure a good rate of growth.

1 1 9

SILICON

Silicon, also known as silica, is the second most plentiful element on the planet after oxygen. It forms long complex molecules, as does carbon, hence its role in plants like bamboo which need to be long, supple, and strong. In humans, silicon is a small but vital trace mineral in all connective tissues, bones, blood vessels, and cartilage. It may have a role in preventing osteoporosis by assisting the utilization of calcium within the bones.

ABOVE A high level of silicon is found in the skin of cucumbers.

The silicon content of the aorta, trachea, lungs, and tendons is particularly high. Silicon in these tissues seems to decline with age and the amount in the arterial walls decreases with the development of atherosclerosis. Silicon also helps strengthen skin, hair, and nails by improving the production of collagen and keratin.

Silicon is required for the proper functioning of an enzyme that assists in the formation of collagen in bone, cartilage, and other connective tissues. It has been found in very high concentrations at the calcification sites in growing bones.

In the absence of a large amount of scientific knowledge about silicon, it is still a popular nutrient recommended for the strengthening of hair, skin, bones, and connective tissue.

DIETARY SOURCES OF SILICON

It has been estimated that approximately 9 to 14mg of silicon are assimilated per day, but most dietary silicon, in the form of silica, remains unabsorbed. In contrast, silicic acid in foods and beverages is absorbed readily. The richest sources of silicon are whole grains, such as brown rice, millet, and oats, sea vegetables (edible seaweeds), cucumbers (skin), and root vegetables. Silicon is also found in hard water and seafood.

LEFT Brown rice is an extremely rich source of silicon, and is an important dietary component.

DIETARY REFERENCE VALUES FOR SILICON

There is no RNI for silicon. Some research suggests that the UK diet provides around 1.2g (1,200mg) per day; a Finnish study suggested that 29mg/day was typical. Other studies suggest levels of around 200mg/day are ingested. American sources state that 20–40mg/day is safe and adequate.

SILICON AND MUSCLE TISSUE

Silicon is a vital trace mineral in all connective tissues.

ABOVE Silicon improves the production of collagen and keratin.

SILICON SUPPLEMENTATION

Silicon is available in several different forms. Silicon-rich plants like horsetail (*Equisetum arvense*) are commonly found as supplements. Others include powdered bamboo gum (*Bambousa arundinacea*), sodium metasilicate, and colloidal silicic acid. The dosages of silica range from 50 to 200mg per capsule and it is occasionally found in multiformulas. The colloidal form can also be used topically in skin-rejuvenating creams.

Silicon is generally regarded as being nontoxic. However, increased levels of silicon and aluminum complexes have been detected in the plaques of brain tissue from Alzheimer's patients, but it is thought that the dietary and environmental sources of aluminum are more significant than the silicon and, in fact, silicon has been suggested as an antagonist against aluminum in the prevention of Alzheimer's disease.

DEFICIENCY SYMPTOMS

WEAKENED NAILS.

POOR SKIN AND HAIR INTEGRITY.

WEAKENED BONES AND TENDONS.

RIGHT Increase your consumption of fresh vegetables to aid your silicon absorption.

CLINICAL REPORT

One of the few studies carried out on colloidal silicic acid was with a group of women with signs of aging of their skin (face), thin hair, and brittle nails. A daily dose of 10 milliliters of colloidal silicic acid was taken orally, and colloidal silicic acid applied topically twice a day. Significant improvements were noted in the thickness and strength of the skin, hair, and nails, and a loss of wrinkles.

BELOW Breakfasting on porridge made from wholegrains gives a good silicon boost to the body.

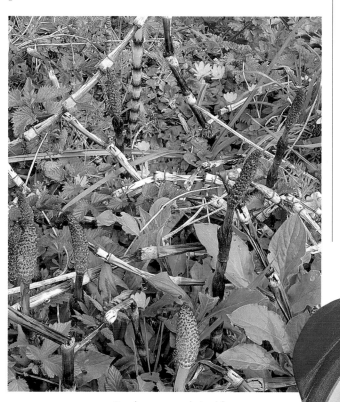

ABOVE Supplements are derived from silicon-rich plants such as horsetail.

FUNCTIONS OF SILICON

- Essential for formation of collagen.

- Essential for healthy bone, cartilage, tendon, and other connective tissues.

- Necessary for healthy skin, hair, and nails.

- Necessary for healthy blood vessels.

- Necessary for healthy trachea and lungs.

- May prevent osteoporosis and atherosclerosis.

VANADIUM

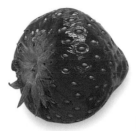

Vanadium is a mineral that has recently received a great deal of attention in medical literature. Its name comes from the Scandinavian goddess of beauty and youth. It was used by French doctors at the turn of the 20th century as a miracle cure for a variety of illnesses, but it lost favor for a time because high dosages caused toxicity.

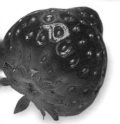

ABOVE **Strawberries are a tasty source of vanadium.**

Most research on vanadium has focused on its role in improving or mimicking the action of insulin. Some studies on animals have shown that vanadyl sulfate led to improved glucose tolerance, inhibition of cholesterol synthesis, and improved mineralization of teeth and bones. Vanadyl sulfate is also popular with bodybuilders.

In-vitro (test tube) and animal studies indicate that vanadium has a specific physiological role in humans as a regulator of the enzyme sodium/potassium-ATPase, and is therefore involved in activity of the sodium/potassium pump mechanism within the membrane of cells. This has yet to be fully proven, but if found to be correct, it may become a helpful biochemical tool for use in regulation of cellular exchanges—the nourishment of cells and the subsequent removal of toxins.

Vanadium may also have a role in methyl metabolism and thereby endocrine function. Unlike some harmful mineral elements like cadmium and lead, vanadium does not accumulate in body tissues with age and its concentrations in serum is minutely small.

VANADIUM CONTENT IN FOOD

It is not known how useful the numerical content figures are, since some research indicates that most ingested vanadium—about 99 percent—is not absorbed. The estimated daily intake of vanadium for American adults is 10–60mcg. Total body content is about 100mcg, but this is not concentrated in any one particular organ or tissue. Good food sources include parsley, lettuce, radish, fresh seed oils, and shellfish. Black pepper is also a good source.

DIETARY REFERENCE VALUES FOR VANADIUM

Dietary requirement has not been well defined as yet. The amount lost in the urine is approximately 10mcg per day; this, then, would seem to be the minimum requirement. However, Dietary Reference Values state that the requirement is possibly only about 1–2mcg per day, while American sources suggest that a daily intake of between 10 and 60mcg is deemed to be safe.

RIGHT **For a daily vanadium boost, eat a crisp mixed salad with a dressing of seed oil.**

DIETARY SOURCES OF VANADIUM MCG/100G					
PARSLEY	2,950	SUNFLOWER OIL	41	CABBAGE	10
LOBSTER	1,610	CUCUMBER	38	GARLIC	10
RADISHES	790	OATS	35	CAULIFLOWER	9
DILL	460	APPLES	33	TOMATOES	6
LETTUCE	280	OLIVE OIL	30	ONIONS	5
BUCKWHEAT	100	SUNFLOWER SEEDS	15	BEET	4
STRAWBERRIES	70	CORN	15	PLUMS	2
SOYBEANS	70	GREEN BEANS	14	MILLET	2
SAFFLOWER OIL	64	PEANUT OIL	11		
SARDINES	46	CARROTS	10		

VANADIUM DEFICIENCY SYMPTOMS

Although vanadium may have a function in hormone processes, cholesterol biochemistry, and blood-sugar metabolism, no specific deficiency symptoms have been reported. Vanadium deficiency may contribute to elevated cholesterol levels, and faulty blood sugar control, leading to hypoglycemia and possibly diabetes.

FUNCTIONS OF VANADIUM

- Involved in glucose metabolism.
- May mimic the action of insulin.
- Involved in the transport (pump) mechanism in cell membranes.
- May be involved in endocrine function.
- Involved in mineralization of bones and teeth.
- May be involved in balancing cholesterol levels.
- May prevent heart attacks and reduce high blood pressure.
- May be involved in detoxification.

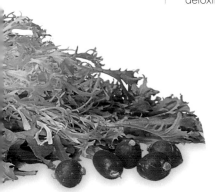

LEFT Lobster has very high levels of vanadium, and is a luxury option for a mineral boost!

VANADIUM SUPPLEMENTATION

Vanadium exists in several different forms with the most biologically active being vanadyl or vanadate; the most popular is vanadyl sulfate. A dosage range of 50 to 100mcg per day should be a safe and sufficient amount to meet nutritional requirements.

Toxic effects of vanadium (in the form of vanadate) from animal studies include elevation of blood pressure, reduction of coenzyme A and coenzyme Q10 levels, stimulation of monoamine oxidase inhibitors, and interference with cellular energy production. There is some evidence that excessive supplementation with vanadium may be linked to manic depression. Vanadium may interfere with lithium, a mineral that is prescribed for manic depression.

High vitamin C levels may reduce the amount of vanadium in the body. Also, vanadium is an antagonist of chromium and may, therefore, reduce chromium levels if taken in excess. Foods high in vanadium are usually low in chromium.

There are no known interactions with vanadium and drugs other than that with lithium.

ZINC

Zinc is one of the most important trace elements in our diet. Along with vitamin C, it is a vital protector of the immune system and an essential mineral for the structure and function of all cell membranes. The beneficial effects of zinc are extensive because of its involvement in so many enzyme reactions and body structures. Adequate levels of zinc are necessary for proper immune function, which means that even a small deficiency can result in an increased susceptibility to infection.

ABOVE One of the most important trace elements, zinc is found in pecans.

It is involved in hundreds of enzyme pathways in which it has structural, regulatory, or catalytic roles, and is found in all body tissues. In addition, it has a structural role in a number of non-enzymic proteins like those involved in insulin production and in genetic transcription. Zinc is involved, then, in the major metabolic pathways leading to the metabolism of proteins, carbohydrates, fats, energy and nucleic acids.

Zinc is found in its highest concentration in the muscles (65 percent of the total), red and white blood cells, bone, skin, liver, kidneys, pancreas, retina of the eyes, and, in males, in the prostate gland and sperm. The adult body contains about 2 to 3g of zinc, which is quite a significant amount. Early features of deficiency include growth retardation, skin problems, loss of integrity of intestinal membranes, and poor immune function.

Zinc occurs in every cell of the body and is a component of over 200 enzymes. It functions in more enzymatically controlled reactions than any other mineral. It is also necessary for the healthy functioning of many body hormones, including thymus hormones, insulin, growth hormone, and sex hormones. It will be obvious, therefore, that zinc is vital for growing children, particularly during puberty when both growth spurts and hormonal activation are important.

Furthermore, because of zinc's importance in skin structure, early teenage males (who are growing rapidly and are also being bombarded with newly emerging sex hormones) are the group most likely to suffer from acne (although teenage girls also suffer from this condition too). The presence of acne in this age range is correlated closely with reduced serum zinc levels.

The maintenance of optimal zinc levels is essential in all age groups for general good health. It is required for protein synthesis and cell growth and, therefore, for wound-healing, especially after surgery or in recovery from burns. It also has an important role in vision, taste, and smell, and this means that a drop in body zinc levels may result in an impairment of these special senses. Night blindness can occur as a result of zinc deficiency in addition to that of vitamin A. Loss of sense of taste and smell is common in the elderly, when zinc absorption can be impaired by the ageing process. Because of zinc's role in male sexual function, a deficiency is a possible factor in the high rate of prostate enlargement and male infertility.

BELOW "Popcorn" contains zinc, essential for growing children

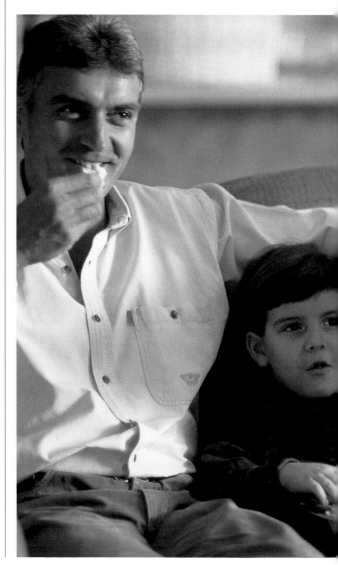

DIETARY SOURCES OF ZINC MG/100G

OYSTERS, FRESH	148.7	RYE	3.2	EGGS	1.5
POPCORN, FRESHLY "POPPED"	8.3	OATS	3.2	TURNIPS	1.2
SESAME SEEDS	7.8	PEANUTS	3.2	CHICKEN	1.1
PUMPKIN SEEDS	7.5	LIMA BEANS	3.1	SOYBEANS, COOKED	1.0
GINGER ROOT	6.8	ALMONDS	3.1	PARSLEY	0.9
CRAB	5.5	WALNUTS	3.0	WHOLE-WHEAT PASTA, BOILED	0.7
PECANS	4.5	LOBSTER, COOKED	3.0	GARLIC	0.6
FIELD PEAS, DRY	4.2	SARDINES, CANNED	2.9	CARROTS	0.5
BRAZIL NUTS	4.2	BUCKWHEAT	2.5	BOSTON BAKED BEANS	0.5
CHEESE, CHEDDAR	4.0	HAZELNUTS	2.4	FISH, WHITE	0.4
BEEF, STEWING STEAK	3.8	BREAD, WHOLE-WHEAT	1.8	POTATOES, OLD	0.3
WHOLE WHEAT	3.2	GREEN PEAS	1.6		

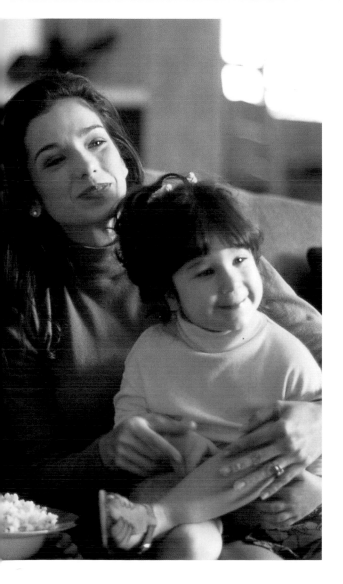

DIETARY REFERENCE VALUES FOR ZINC

	rni mg/day	rda mg/day
0–6 MONTHS	4.0	5 (under 1 year)
7 MONTHS TO 3 YEARS	5.0	10 (1 – 10 years)
4–6 YEARS	6.5	10
7–10 YEARS	7.0	10
11–14 YEARS	9.0	(males) 15 (females 12)
15+ YEARS (MALES)	9.5	15
15+ YEARS (FEMALES)	7.0	12
PREGNANCY	7.0	15
LACTATION (0–4 MONTHS)	13.0	19
LACTATION (4 + MONTHS)	9.5	19

RIGHT Crunchy pumpkin seeds are a good source of zinc.

ZINC CONTENT IN FOOD

The most well-known food source for zinc is oysters, but it is present in fairly high amounts in other shellfish, fish, and red meats. Moderate to good amounts are found in several plant foods such as seeds (especially pumpkin and sesame), nuts, pulses, and whole grains. However, zinc from plant sources is, like iron, less available. It binds to

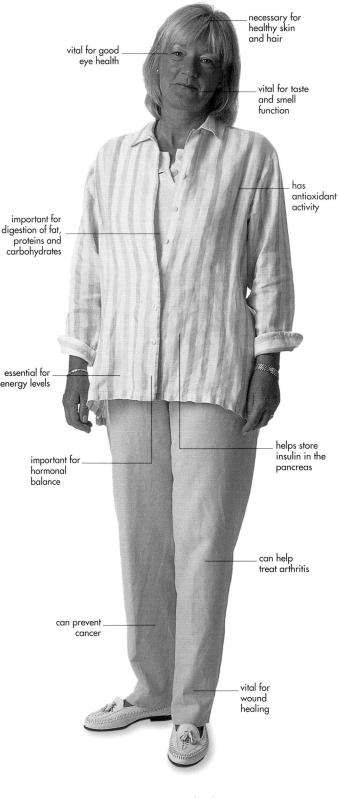

necessary for
healthy skin
and hair

vital for good
eye health

vital for taste
and smell
function

has
antioxidant
activity

important for
digestion of fat,
proteins and
carbohydrates

essential for
energy levels

important for
hormonal
balance

helps store
insulin in the
pancreas

can help
treat arthritis

can prevent
cancer

vital for
wound
healing

ABOVE Zinc is essential to the structure
and function of all cell membranes.

FUNCTIONS OF ZINC

- Essential for growth.

- Involved in over 200 enzymic reactions.

- Vital for immune function.

- Essential for genetic transcription and metabolism of nucleic acids.

- Necessary for cell membrane structure and function.

- Necessary for healthy skin and intestinal lining.

- Necessary for eye health.

- Has antioxidant activity.

- Important for the prostate gland.

- Important for sperm production.

- Important for hormonal activity.

- Required for prostaglandin synthesis.

- Involved in the storage of insulin in the pancreas.

- Important for metabolism of proteins, carbohydrates, and fats.

- Important for production of energy.

- Involved in detoxification.

- Necessary for vitamin A metabolism.

- Necessary for the synthesis of collagen.

- Involved in the mechanism of taste and smell.

- Required for efficient wound-healing.

- Prevents cancer.

- May help in degenerative conditions.

- Is used therapeutically in the treatment of male infertility and poor sexual function, acne, anorexia, mouth ulcers, viral infections, herpes, poor immune function, sickle-cell anemia, tinnitus, thyroid conditions, arthritis, ulcers, growth problems, cancer, allergies, alcoholic cirrhosis, Alzheimer's disease, general inflammatory conditions, macular degeneration, night blindness.

phytic acid (a compound in fiber) and forms zinc-phytate which is not absorbed. Since seeds and nuts are lower in fiber than whole grain cereals and pulses, seeds and nuts are an ideal source of zinc for vegans and vegetarians, and at the same time provide many essential fatty acids.

Zinc turnover in body tissues is slow and stores of zinc in the body do not provide a reliable source at times of deprivation. Thus, the body is dependent on a regular dietary supply of zinc. Zinc is absorbed throughout the gut, but a major part of it is absorbed in the distal part of the small intestine. Zinc competes for absorption with other minerals, especially calcium, iron, and copper, so that high intakes of these minerals, can adversely affect zinc absorption. The Western diet is generally very high in calcium, principally from dairy foods, and low in zinc.

ABOVE Meat-eaters will obtain a plentiful supply of zinc from stewing steak.

Compounded with this is the (often misleading) advice for many sections of the population to take calcium supplements without supplementation of the other minerals, notably zinc and magnesium. Drinking tea or coffee with meals inhibits the absorption of zinc.

CONDITIONS RELATED TO DECREASED ZINC INTAKE

ACUTE INFECTIONS	INFLAMMATION
AGING	PROTEIN DEFICIENCY
ALCOHOLISM	VEGETARIANISM
ANOREXIA NERVOSA	WEIGHT-LOSS DIETS (AND FAD DIETS IN GENERAL)
INCREASED LOSS FROM BODY (BURNS, POST-TRAUMA, STARVATION)	

CONDITIONS RELATED TO POOR ABSORPTION OF ZINC

ALCOHOLISM	LIVER DISEASE
CELIAC DISEASE	LOW STOMACH ACID (HYPOCHLORHYDRIA)
DIARRHEA	
EXCESS INTAKE OF CALCIUM	PANCREATIC INSUFFICIENCY
EXCESS INTAKE OF IRON	POOR BLOOD-SUGAR BALANCE (AND HYPOGLYCEMIA, DIABETES)
HIGH-FIBER DIET	
INFLAMMATORY BOWEL DISORDERS	

CLINICAL REPORTS

IMMUNE FUNCTION

Zinc is intimately involved with immunity. When zinc levels are low, white cells (T-cells) are lower in number, the functioning of all types of white cell is greatly impaired, and hormones from the thymus gland are reduced. Zinc supplementation dramatically reverses these trends. Also zinc possesses direct antiviral activity and can therefore be effective against the common cold virus. A double-blind study demonstrated that zinc-containing lozenges significantly reduced the average length of colds by seven days. After the seven-day period was concluded, over 80 percent of the zinc-supplemented patients were symptom-free as opposed to less than half of the placebo-treated patients.

MALE SEXUAL FUNCTION

Zinc functions in almost every aspect of male reproduction—testosterone production, sperm formation, sperm motility, potency. One typical piece of research studied men who had suffered infertility for five years or more. Some of these subjects had very low sperm counts and poor blood levels of testosterone. The men received a supplement containing 60mg of zinc daily for around six weeks. In over half the men with low testosterone levels, average sperm count more than doubled, along with a marked increase in the amounts of testosterone.

ALZHEIMER'S DISEASE

Zinc deficiency is probably the most common deficiency in elderly individuals and since zinc is involved in so many cellular functions, it may be that dementia is associated with accumulation of genetic and metabolic errors in a low zinc environment in the tissues.

Moreover, since zinc is involved in many antioxidant enzyme functions, prolonged low zinc levels may result in the destruction of nerve tissue due to free-radical damage. The levels of zinc in the brain and spinal fluid of Alzheimer's patients have been found to be significantly lower than those suffering no dementia. There is some evidence that zinc supplementation can improve memory, communication, and social interaction in some Alzheimer's sufferers.

CLINICAL DEFICIENCY SYMPTOMS

ALCOHOL ABUSE

ABNORMAL MENSTRUATION

ANOREXIA

BEHAVIORAL PROBLEMS

CONNECTIVE TISSUE DISORDERS

DELAYED WOUND HEALING

DELAYED SEXUAL MATURATION

DEPRESSION

FREQUENT SEVERE INFECTIONS

GROWTH RETARDATION

IMPAIRED GLUCOSE

TOLERANCE

IMPOTENCE

INFERTILITY

INFLAMMATORY BOWEL DISEASE

MALABSORPTION SYNDROMES

NIGHT BLINDNESS

PSYCHIATRIC ILLNESS

RHEUMATOID ARTHRITIS

SEVERE SKIN CONDITIONS (ACNE, ECZEMA, PSORIASIS)

SLEEP DISTURBANCES

UNUSUAL HAIR LOSS

MILD DEFICIENCY SYMPTOMS

WHITE SPOTS ON FINGERNAILS (POOR HEALING SECONDARY TO NAIL TRAUMA)

WHITE COATING ON TONGUE

MARKED HALITOSIS

HAIR LOSS (OR VERY SLOW TO GROW)

DANDRUFF

STRETCH MARKS

POOR APPETITE

DETERIORATING SENSE OF TASTE AND SMELL

POOR IMMUNE FUNCTION

POOR SKIN

DEFICIENCY SYMPTOMS

Severe zinc deficiency is rare in developed countries but many individuals in the United States, Britain and other parts of the Western world have marginal zinc deficiency. Groups most at risk are the elderly, young teenagers (especially males), pregnant and breastfeeding women, and vegans and vegetarians. Zinc deficiency may also be high in those taking the contraceptive pill or HRT, and in those suffering from chronic illnesses such as arthritis and rheumatism.

BELOW Zinc is found in seeds, nuts, pulses, and whole grains.

ABOVE Young developing males are at risk from zinc deficiency, and may need extra supplementation.

ZINC SUPPLEMENTATION

There are many forms of zinc supplements—zinc sulfate, zinc picolinate, zinc acetate, zinc citrate, zinc glycerate, zinc monomethionine, zinc chelates. Most of these forms are well absorbed. Some evidence shows that zinc citrate is very well absorbed since it is the form that is found in human breast milk.

The dosage range for zinc supplementation for general health support is 15–20mg per day. When zinc supplementation is used to address specific needs (always under the supervision of a practitioner or physician), the dosage range increases to 30–60mg/day for men and 30–45mg/day for women. Long-term supplementation with zinc requires that vitamin B6, selenium, and copper are also supplemented. Zinc competes with copper for absorption, and other minerals (calcium and iron) can adversely affect zinc absorption if supplemented at a high dosage. Zinc supplements need to be taken with food, since nausea will occur if taken on an empty stomach. Also, zinc supplements should be taken at a different time in the day from high-fiber foods for maximum absorption of zinc. Zinc does not appear to interact in a negative way with any drug.

ABOVE By far the greatest concentration of zinc is found in oysters.

Zinc is considered to be nontoxic, at moderate levels. Very high doses (above 150mg/day), or lower doses for prolonged periods of time, may produce copper-induced anemia, interference with iron metabolism, reduced HDL cholesterol (good cholesterol) levels, and depressed immune function.

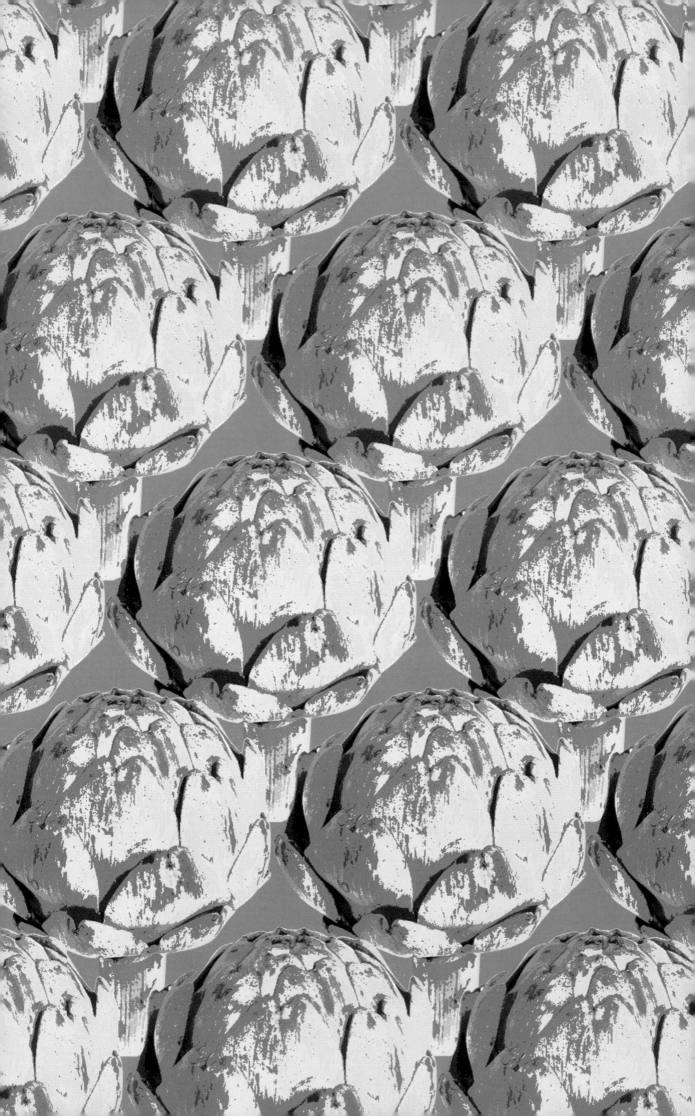

PART FOUR

OPTIMIZING YOUR DIET

Everyone would like to lead a long and healthy life, free from pain and illness, and the careful use of nutritional substances can help us go some way to achieving this goal. Vitamins and minerals can act to ensure the optimum functioning of all the organs and systems in our body. They are now known to boost immunity, stimulate our mental performance, extend our lives, and prevent serious health problems, such as heart diseases, immune conditions, and cancer. People of any age can benefit from the prudent use of nutritional therapy, and there are special treatment programs designed for babies, pregnant women, children, the elderly, and those with serious health problems.

INCREASE YOUR ENERGY LEVELS

At least 50 percent of adults seeking medical treatment complain of some form of fatigue. It may be constant, beginning upon waking even after a full night's sleep, or it may build during the day until by evening you feel utterly exhausted. Even very light exercise may cause extreme tiredness, or bouts of fatigue may seem to occur after eating or drinking a specific food or beverage. The number of patients complaining of being permanently tired is increasing; so much so that the symptom now has an acronym—TAT (tired all the time).

Though fatigue may be due to an underlying condition, often no evidence of another illness can be found. Several studies indicate that a large number of cases of "chronic" fatigue are caused by: food intolerance; excessive intakes of caffeine, sugar, and refined carbohydrate or high GI (glycemic index) foods; toxicity of the body; or multiple deficiencies.

ABOVE Eat basmati brown rice instead of processed white rice for energy.

BELOW Exercise should leave you feeling refreshed, not exhausted.

FOOD INTOLERANCE

Food intolerance has been implicated in the cause of "allergic tension–fatigue syndrome" consisting of bouts of hyperactivity and fatigue along with classical allergy symptoms, such as asthma or headaches. The foods most associated with sensitivity are wheat, cow's milk, eggs, and citrus, though almost any food eaten regularly could be the culprit. An elimination diet may be needed to remove the offending foods. You could try some detective work yourself and keep a food and symptom diary for a few weeks. At the end of this period, several foods may appear as possible culprits, and you might try leaving these out of your diet for a few weeks to see what happens. Unlike true allergies, however, intolerance symptoms to food can take anything up to 72 hours to develop, which makes relating food to symptom very difficult. You could simply cut out the main food allergens—wheat, and so on—one by one for a period of a few weeks and see how you feel, and then try reintroducing them one at a time.

Alternatively, try a hypoallergenic diet where all potential allergens are omitted. You might try this diet for two or three weeks and, if most of your symptoms have abated, try reintroducing the foods—one food every three or four days. Any food to which you are sensitive will cause a return of symptoms within three days.

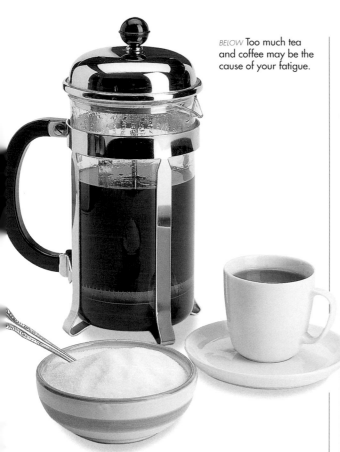

BELOW Too much tea and coffee may be the cause of your fatigue.

The high carbohydrate diet, advocated by many as the answer to reducing the amount of fat and protein, seems now to be a possible cause of imbalanced pancreatic function and insulin insensitivity in some individuals. This imbalance may be severe enough to be a cause of obesity, heart disease, and diabetes and is certainly a contender for food-related fatigue.

HYPOALLERGENIC DIET

- Omit all gluten-containing grains (wheat, rye, oats, barley)—eat brown rice (especially basmati), quinoa, popcorn, polenta, buckwheat, millet.
- Omit all dairy produce (milk [cow's, goat's, or sheep's], cheese, cream, butter, yogurt made from animal milks) and eggs—have soy milk, rice milk, hazelnut milk, coconut milk, soy cheese, soy margarine, live soy yogurt.
- Omit all yeast-containing foods and beverages: yeast extract, breads, fermented products vinegar, wine.
- Omit all citrus fruit (oranges, lemons, grapefruit, tangerines, mandarins, clementines—have any other type of fruit instead.
- Omit all sugar—a little honey or dried fruit can be used for sweetening cereals.
- Omit all food additives (processed and refined food).

CAFFEINE AND REFINED CARBOHYDRATES

Although caffeine can quickly relieve fatigue and increase endurance, chronic caffeine use, especially at high levels of intake, is a hidden cause of fatigue. Since caffeine gives an initial energy boost but at the same time is a metabolic cause of fatigue, a vicious circle is soon established in which increasing amounts of caffeine are needed to prevent withdrawal fatigue. Also, white sugar has long been suspected of promoting fatigue when consumed at high levels, despite its obvious initial energy high. Not only sugar, but other refined or "concentrated" carbohydrates, such as rice, may have this effect. Carbohydrates promote the synthesis of serotonin, a calming neurotransmitter, in the brain which then brings on a feeling of sleepiness. If you suspect caffeine or refined/concentrated carbohydrates as being the cause of your fatigue, the only solution is to remove them from the diet and replace them with a low-caffeine/low carbohydrate substitute. For example, use grain or dandelion root coffee, or Rooibosch tea. Cut out sugar altogether, but don't make the mistake of using artificial sweeteners, since these have problems of their own and in any case are no solution if you are trying to wean yourself off sweet tastes. Wholegrain carbohydrates can be substituted for refined types—brown rice instead of white; whole-wheat pasta instead of white; whole-grain bread instead of white. But, even these "healthier" types of carbohydrate need to be balanced properly with protein and fat.

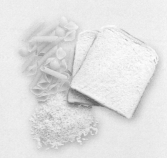

Brown basmati rice, popcorn, and polenta are all excellent foods to eat when you are attempting a hypoallergenic diet.

Avoid overprocessed foods, such as white bread, white pasta, and white flour. These will only exacerbate any sensitivities you have.

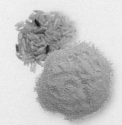

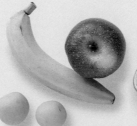

Non-citrus fruit, such as apples, apricots, and bananas, are the best kinds to eat on this type of diet, and are less harsh.

Citrus fruits are a common irritant for most people, and should be omitted immediately when you start this hypoallergenic diet.

133

SOME EXAMPLES FROM THE GLYCEMIC INDEX		
HIGH GI FOODS	MODERATE GI FOODS	LOW GI FOODS
COOKED PARSNIPS	RYE BREAD AND CRISPBREAD	OATMEAL PORRIDGE
COOKED CARROTS	UNSWEETENED MUESLI	BOSTON BAKED BEANS (NO SUGAR)
BOILED WHITE RICE	BROWN LONG GRAIN RICE	DRIED PEAS
BAKED POTATO	COOKED BEETS	SWEET POTATO
CORNFLAKES	BOILED NEW POTATOES	WHOLE-WHEAT SPAGHETTI
WHEAT-BASED CEREALS	BANANA (NOT SWEET)	APPLE JUICE
BAGELS	CORN AND POLENTA	ORANGES
PUFFED RICE CEREAL	BASMATI RICE	WAX BEANS
RICE CAKES	SULTANAS	GARBANZO BEANS
CORN CHIPS	OATMEAL COOKIES	APPLES, PEARS
BEAN CURD ICE CREAM	ORANGE JUICE	ICE CREAM (FULL-FAT)
WHEAT BREAD	GARDEN PEAS	WHOLE MILK
MANGO	BUCKWHEAT	BLACK-EYE PEAS
PAPAYA	WHITE SPAGHETTI	KIDNEY BEANS
BANANA (FULLY RIPE)	PINTO BEANS	LENTILS, SOYBEANS

LEFT Include a range of whole grains in your diet—rice, oats, wheat, and barley.

BELOW Balance your carbohydrates with protein foods.

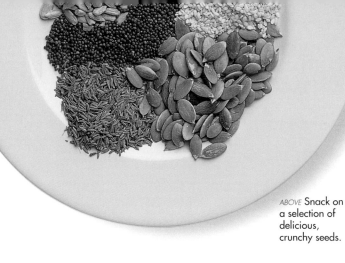
ABOVE Snack on a selection of delicious, crunchy seeds.

GLYCEMIC INDEX

Carbohydrates of all types have been tested to assess how quickly they are able to release glucose into the blood (and stimulate insulin production). From this, a Glycemic Index of foods has been drawn up, relating each food to pure glucose. Old favorites, such as baked potato and white rice, are high on this list. If your diet contains many such "high GI" foods, then these need to be reduced or balanced with protein.

TOXINS

If your lifestyle exposes you to a large number of toxins, perhaps in the form of pollution, smoking, food additives, pesticides or excessive intake of alcohol, then your body will be working hard to remove these from the body. Detoxification uses a lot of energy; it is essential that you take steps to deal with as many of these sources as possible, by eliminating processed foods, drinking plenty of water, oxygenating your system through exercise and making other lifestyle changes where this is possible.

A distinct possibility for the causative agent of fatigue is a nutrient deficiency (or multiple micronutrient deficiency). Many minerals and vitamins work together to control and maintain the release of energy from foods. The B vitamins, vitamin C, iron, magnesium, zinc, copper, manganese, and germanium are all involved

in this process. It follows, then, that a deficiency in any one of these micronutrients is going to slow the process of metabolism down and, in so doing, cause fatigue. To improve the intake of these essential nutrients you need to include the following in your diet:

• Whole grains—brown basmati rice, quinoa, buckwheat, oats and oatmeal, rye, wheat germ, couscous, cracked wheat, pot barley, popped corn.
• Lean meat and poultry, or fish, or dark green vegetables, or pulses.
• Plenty of fresh vegetables (including garlic) and fruit—a good color mix.
• Seeds, fresh—sesame, sunflower, pumpkin, and flaxseeds.
• Nuts, fresh –Brazils, almonds, walnuts, cashews.
• A good quality multiformula supplement, including vitamin C (500–1000mg/day), all the B vitamins, magnesium, iron, copper, manganese, potassium, and zinc.

RIGHT Fresh, mixed nuts are a good source of several nutrients
.
BELOW Take a good quality multiformula supplement every day.

BOVE Fresh vegetables and fruit are healthy and pleasing to the eye.

PREVENT CANCER

Cancer is life-threatening because abnormal cells grow uncontrollably, spreading throughout the body and damaging normal functioning. It is not a single disease with only one cause, but covers more than a hundred malignancies attacking different organs, and has multifactorial causes. Cancer is the second most common killer disease; one out of three people will be diagnosed with it in their lifetimes.

ABOVE Garlic is known to be full of health-sustaining properties.

Around 50 percent, or even more, of cancers are believed to be associated with nutritional factors, especially breast and uterine cancer, prostate cancer, and gastrointestinal cancer. Dietary components implicated in the main are excess fat, low fiber, poor intake of dark green and orange vegetables (low intake of phytochemicals, especially antioxidants), excess sugar, alcohol, some tap waters, and nutrient deficiencies.

FAT

Fat intake has been repeatedly found in studies to be related to the risk of cancer. Many of the studies have implicated saturated fat as the biggest problem. Conversely, a small, daily amount of essential fatty acids from "good" fats found in fresh wholefoods, and particularly seeds, nuts, and fish, are vital for the proper functioning of those systems that will prevent cancer— the immune and hormonal systems.

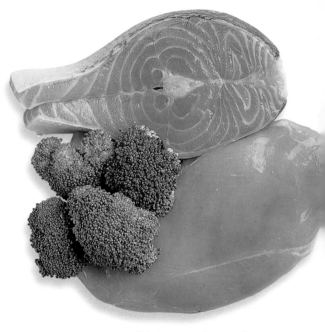

ABOVE Eat fish, lean meat, bean curd, and vegetables to avoid a high intake of saturated fats.

FIBER

The higher your intake of dietary fiber, the lower you risk of cancer, since a high-fiber diet will ensure tha dietary and metabolic toxins (including excess sex ho mones) and cholesterol are removed efficiently from th gut, before these can be reabsorbed in the color However, all fibers are not equal; wheat fiber is a poo choice because it is insoluble and harsh and may irritat the gut lining. Furthermore, wheat fiber can combin with important minerals and carry them out of the body Thus, eating large amounts of wholewheat bread an pasta is not the best way to increase fiber in your diet, bu instead choose a much larger variety of high-fiber food: Eat plenty of whole grains which contain more solubl fiber, such as brown rice, buckwheat, oats; fibrous veg etables and fruits like green beans and strawberrie which contain lignin; and fruits and vegetable containing cellulose, hemicelluloses, mucilage and pectins, found in apples, carrots, broccol oatmeal, and flaxseed.

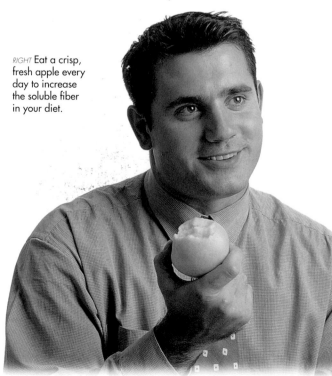

RIGHT Eat a crisp, fresh apple every day to increase the soluble fiber in your diet.

PHYTOCHEMICALS

By increasing your fiber intake, especially from fresh vegetables and fruit, you will also be helping yourself to many of the new-found phytochemicals. These make up hundreds of different important natural substances classified into several different chemical groups, including antioxidants, which have been found to have profound health benefits, by preventing oxidative damage to tissues. Most phytochemicals are important in cancer prevention for a variety of reasons; some optimize immune function, some have a detoxifying effect, some attack free radicals, and others are able to prevent carcinogens from being formed in the gut. Smoked, pickled, and salt-cured foods produce, in the gut, nitrosamines and other substances that are carcinogenic and linked statistically with esophageal and stomach cancers. Phytochemicals can prevent the cancer-causing effect of these foods, and antioxidants can protect against the free radicals that are produced by barbecuing and other food treatments.

All vegetables and fruits, and other foods such as pulses, are likely to contain phytochemicals, but those that have been most researched are as follows: Brassicas (broccoli, cabbage), herbs (especially parsley), dark orange or red foods (carrots, sweet potatoes, tomatoes, hot peppers, apricots, mango), sea vegetables, garlic, fruits (strawberries, citrus, rhubarb, grapes, pineapple, raspberries, blackcurrants), pulses (especially soy), and mushrooms (especially shiitake).

LEFT Rhubarb contains phytochemicals and is high in soluble fiber.

SUGAR AND ALCOHOL

Sugar intake has been shown in several studies to increase the death rate from some cancers. A high sugar intake has been related to an increased risk of breast and colorectal cancers. Research has shown that when healthy people were given additional sugar in their diets, intestinal transit time decreased while the amount of fecal bile acids increased—important changes which can be associated with an increased risk of colorectal cancer.

Alcohol intake, even when modest, is associated with an increased risk of breast cancer, and there is some evidence of an association with other cancers as well.

ABOVE Sweet potatoes are a good source of phytochemicals.

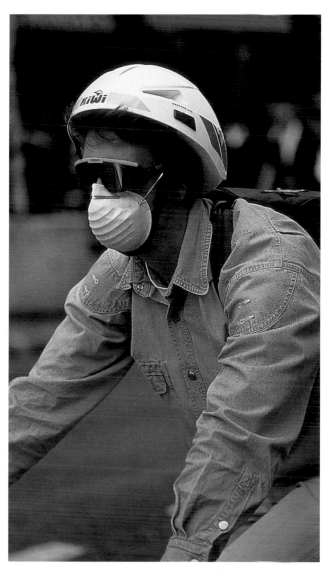

ABOVE Wear a protective mask to avoid inhaling traffic fumes.

DRINKING WATER

Even the hardness of your drinking water affects your risk of getting cancer; the hardness of water is related to dissolved calcium and magnesium. Soft water is acidic, so cadmium and other toxic elements may be leached from pipes in soft water areas, causing them to appear in higher levels in the drinking water. In hard water areas, not only are there lower levels of toxic elements in the drinking water but, due to competition from calcium and magnesium ions, the absorption of toxic elements in the intestines is reduced. The harder your drinking water, the lower your risk of getting cancers of the digestive tract. Note too that chlorination of drinking water (to kill germs) may not be entirely without risk. Bladder cancer has been related to chlorinated drinking water. Also, there is now some concern about the activity of fluoride in those waters that have been artificially fluoridated. If you are concerned about your tap water, the best advice is to use one of the many types of water filter now available or drink bottled spring water. However, natural mineral water is not without its dangers; some have high concentrations of sodium, for example, so ensure you use a range of bottled waters, not just one type.

NUTRIENT DEFICIENCIES

To keep the cancer-preventing systems in good working order, all essential nutrients need to be supplied in optimum amounts. Those deficiencies most implicated in cancer are of: vitamin A, B vitamins (especially B1, B6, and B12), folic acid, choline/inositol, vitamins C, D, and E, calcium, potassium, copper, iron, germanium, molybdenum, selenium, and zinc.

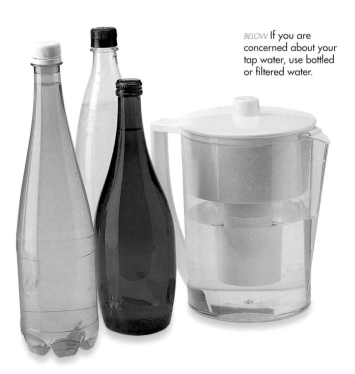

BELOW **If you are concerned about your tap water, use bottled or filtered water.**

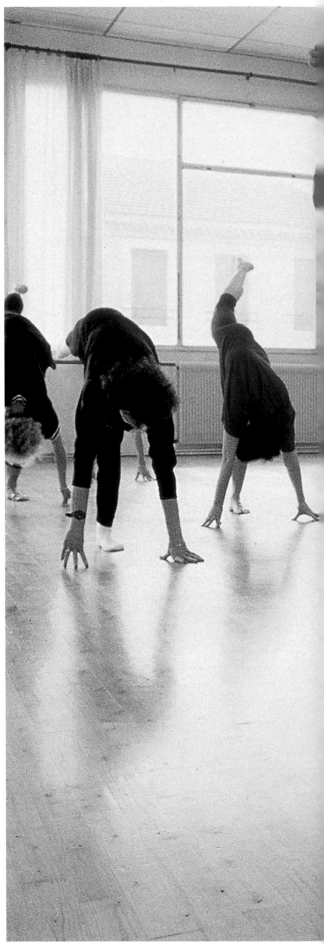

ABOVE **Include regular exercise as part of your anti-cancer lifestyle plan.**

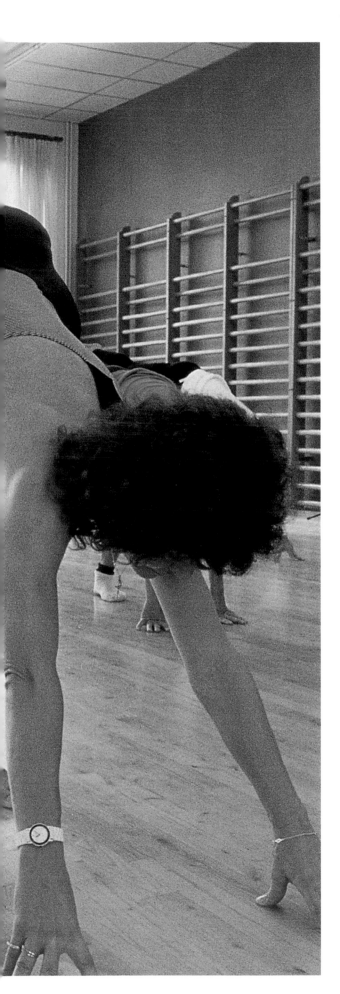

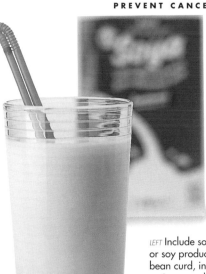

LEFT Include soy milk, or soy products like bean curd, in your anti-cancer diet.

SUPPLEMENTS TO PREVENT CANCER (DAILY DOSAGES)

• A balanced calcium and magnesium supplement: 500mg calcium, 250mg magnesium.
• A multimineral complex containing copper, iron, molybdenum, selenium, and zinc (the amounts will vary, but choose one with good levels of selenium and zinc).
• Vitamin B complex: individual amounts of different B vitamins vary.
• Antioxidant multivitamin (A, C, and E): individual amounts vary.
• Vitamin C: 250 to 500mg two or three times a day.
• Beta-carotene: 25,000 to 45,000IU.
• Vitamin E: 400 to 600IU.

STEPS TO PREVENT CANCER

• Avoid as much saturated fat as possible, but eat foods containing essential fatty acids – seeds, nuts, and oily fish.
• Avoid sugar and over-processed, refined foods.
• Avoid smoked, cured, salted, and barbecued food.
• Cut down on alcohol.
• Eat plenty of fiber in its various forms.
• Eat at least five servings of vegetables and fruit daily; include all the colors (for maximum intake of phytochemicals and potassium).
• Eat garlic regularly (for its excellent antioxidant properties and germanium).
• Drink soy milk, or eat bean curd, three or four times a week.
• Use a water filter or a range of different bottled waters.
• Make other sensible lifestyle changes; stop smoking, take care in the sun (some sun is needed for formation of vitamin D); exercise

LIVE LONGER

An enormous amount of research work has been undertaken on aging and how to delay it. While experts are still not clear about why we age, they do know what causes some of the problems normally associated with aging, and it is therefore possible for us to start to do something about these.

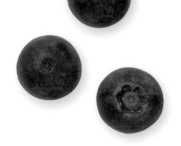

ABOVE Dark blue or purple fruits contain antioxidants.

Damaging free radicals are now considered to be an important factor in aging: formation of wrinkles; balding and other hair changes; the general slowing down of the metabolism; and the tendency towards degenerate illnesses like arthritis, heart disease, diabetes, and cancer. There are also other visible signs, such as decline in height and shrinkage of muscle mass, as well as not-so-visible signs, such as progressive loss of brain and kidney cells and changes in other vital organs—all these are related to poor cell repair and replacement. The regenerating machinery, and particularly the replication of DNA, becomes more and more error-prone as we get older. Many of these internal changes are reflected in the decline of body functions including memory, concentration, hearing, sight, immunity, and circulation.

DIET

Optimizing your diet is the best way to slow down the clock, or even to make it go back a little. Include plenty of nutrient-dense food such as whole grains, vegetables and fruit, seeds, nuts, fish, lean meat, and pulses. All refined and processed food needs to be avoided or reduced to a minimum, and as much produce as possible should be organic. Saturated fats are to be avoided and dairy foods (except live yogurt) need to be restricted, as do sugar and refined carbohydrates.

Since metabolic rate slows generally as we age, the calorific content of our diet needs to reduce gradually, otherwise the result will be clearly visible as extra weight. It need not be grim—you can still have treats as long as your basic diet is high in essential nutrients.

BELOW Make a few lifestyle changes to slow down the aging process.

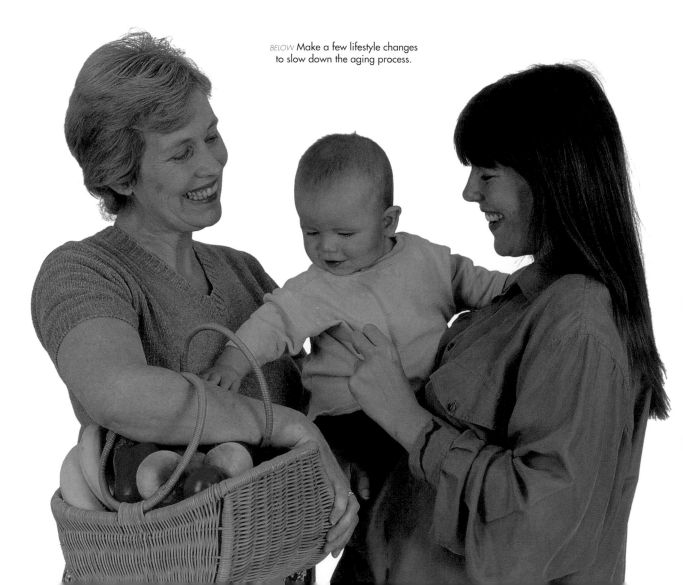

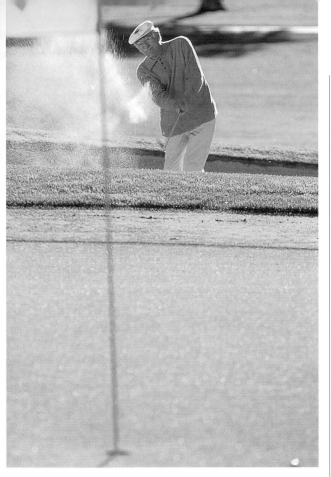

ABOVE Take up a new hobby to stimulate the mind—it'll help you stay younger longer.

ANTIOXIDANTS

To prevent the damaging effect caused by free radicals, a diet high in antioxidants (vitamins A, C, E and minerals such as selenium) is clearly beneficial; these are readily obtained from vegetables, fruits, and whole grains. To ensure your diet includes these antioxidants, and other important phytochemicals, choose a good color mix of vegetables and fruit each day. Vegetables and fruits that are dark green, orange, red, yellow, white, and purple contain plentiful amounts of vitamins A and C and other antioxidants; while a good mixture of wholegrain cereals will supply you with vitamin E. Many other foods, like fresh seeds and nuts, contain a good proportion of antioxidant minerals. Brazil nuts, for example, are high in selenium. Of particular importance are the dark blue/purple fruits like blackcurrants and blueberries. These are a good source of antho-cyanidins (another groups of phytochemicals) that, among a myriad of other benefits, are excellent for maintaining healthy eyes and eyesight.

STEPS TO DELAY THE SIGNS OF AGING

• Eat plenty of leafy green and brightly colored vegetables and fruit.

• Eat antioxidant foods to boost immune function (to build resistance to infection and prevent cancer) and fight free-radical activity (to prevent wrinkles, joint problems, and heart disease).

• Ensure your diet contains a suitable range of fibrous foods for a healthy colon; brown rice, oats, buckwheat, green beans, apples, carrots.

• Eat live yogurt three or four times a week to ensure a healthy gut flora.

• Eat plenty of fresh garlic to stimulate immune function and aid the circulation.

• Avoid saturated fats which clog arteries and add extra weight; instead, have a little olive oil, a mixture of freshly ground mixed seeds, nuts, and fish oils.

• Drink plenty of water (filtered or bottled) to rehydrate your skin and all of your body cells and to flush out toxins.

• Try to avoid a lot of negative stress; stress produces damaging free-radicals.

• Use a good moisturizing cream with a sunscreen; sunshine is important for the production of vitamin D, but too much will cause premature wrinkling of the skin.

• Continue to exercise as you get older; a brisk walk in the fresh air for 20 minutes a day may be all you need, and weight-bearing activity will help ward off osteoporosis and encourage proper circulation and oxygenation of the tissues.

• Do some deep breathing exercises daily to ensure a good intake of oxygen.

• Take up a hobby—a stimulated mind will always be a young mind.

• Make other lifestyle changes—avoid smoking and smoky atmospheres; cut down on alcohol; relax properly, but save your sleeping for night time.

• Take any good quality multiformula supplement daily; ensure it contains beta-carotene, vitamins C, E, and the B complex, selenium, zinc, calcium, magnesium, iron, manganese, and silica.

LEFT Eating fresh fruits helps prevent free radical damage.

ACHIEVE YOUR NATURAL WEIGHT

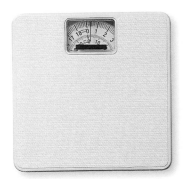

Being overweight can be uncomfortable, especially in hot weather. It can lead to serious health problems such as heart disease, diabetes, and cancer. For most people, though, overweight is something that makes us very unhappy, almost to the extent of feeling an outcast from society. This poor self-image itself can lead to ill health.

LEFT Aim to lose weight at a rate of no more than 2lb (1kg) a week.

The first step to losing weight is to be sensible about what is possible. The perfect shape is unattainable for most of us; so is losing half a stone a week. It has been said over and over again, but nevertheless it is true, that weight loss needs to occur at around one to two pounds a week, otherwise more water and muscle will be lost in preference to fat.

METABOLIC RATE

The amount of "lean body mass" (muscle tissue) is crucial to a healthy metabolic rate. The higher the amount of muscle tissue, the faster the metabolism of the whole body will be because muscle tissue is much more demanding of energy than fat. This is why men find losing weight easier than women—their ratio of muscle to fat is higher. Lose muscle mass and you lose the ability to lose fat! This is clearly seen in the so called "yo-yo" dieters who lose weight (water, muscle, and fat) but gain the whole lot back again, plus a little more each time. The reason for this is that lean muscle tissue has been lost. The weight returning is almost all fat and metabolism will be consequently slower. It then becomes even more difficult to lose weight.

EXERCISE

The second step to losing weight is to improve blood flow to the muscles (to supply nutrients and oxygen) and encourage healthy metabolism therein. This is of paramount importance to any weight loss program and we do it by exercising. It doesn't need to be overstrenuous but it does need to be continuous for about 30 minutes a day; that is, it needs to be aerobic exercise. A good brisk walk in the fresh air each day, or a swimming session, or a low-impact aerobics class, is sufficient to increase muscle mass. This amount of exercise will not build weigh-lifters' type muscles, but you should notice an increase in strength and energy levels.

BELOW Try to stay in the recommended weight limits for your height, age, and build.

NUTRIENTS

The third step involves supplying the correct nutrients to improve those muscles and get them to burn the fat. There does not need to be any calorie counting, fat counting, deprivation, or self-denial—these approaches tend to produce an obsessiveness or fear of food, and in any case are rarely effective in long-term weight loss. Furthermore, if calorie restriction is severe, the body gets the "famine" message and hangs on to fat even more by reducing metabolic rate. This does not mean that you can eat everything in sight, however, even healthy food; it means listening carefully to your body and feeding it nourishing, strengthening food, when it is hungry. No eating just because food looks nice, or it's meal time, or any other excuse for putting food in your mouth apart from when you feel that tummy-rumbling hunger.

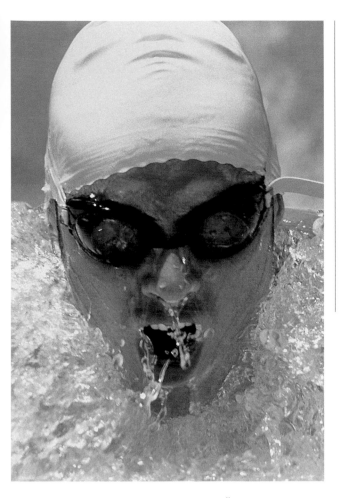

ABOVE Fast swimming is an excellent form of aerobic exercise.

BELOW Keeping a record of your inch-loss will encourage you to keep going.

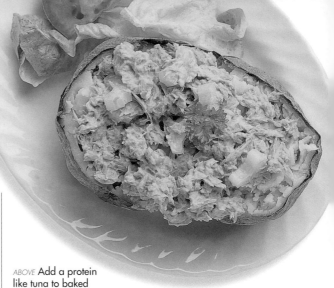

STEPS TO ACHIEVE YOUR NATURAL WEIGHT

• Follow the "thirds" idea to balance the macronutrients and obtain all the essential micronutrients. Fruit and vegetables can be eaten on their own if required.

• Eat whole-grain carbohydrates, not refined processed ones, to balance blood-sugar and supply fiber.

• Eat mainly the low to moderate GI carbohydrates to feel energetic.

• Eat only when you are truly hungry; some of us still confuse mouth hunger with real hunger—try to understand the difference.

• Try not to eat your largest meal in the evening and in any case do not eat after around 8pm, unless you have a little fresh fruit.

• Enjoy your food; eat a basic nutrient-dense diet with a few treats now and again.

• Drink around six medium-sized glasses of water to flush out toxins; the body tends to store its toxins in our fat, so that as you lose fat, toxins are released into the blood.

• Instead of tea and coffee, drink ginger or cinnamon tea; heat-producing herbs can temporarily raise metabolism, albeit slightly— every little helps.

• Take a daily good quality multiformula containing all essential micronutrients; ensure that your multiformula contains chromium and all the B complex of vitamins (including folic acid, biotin, choline, and inositol). If your thyroid gland needs a little boost, try taking some kelp or other sea vegetable in soups and stews (also ensure your multiformula contains zinc and selenium).

• For six days out of seven, do 30 minutes gentle aerobic exercise and try using a few hand weights to increase muscle tone.

• Try to stand and sit correctly; improved posture can make you look thinner instantly.

• Wear clothes that are correct for your present size, or even a slightly larger size for the time being; tight clothes only draw the eye to all the bulges.

• Get sufficient rest and relaxation; when you are feeling rested, your sense of well-being will improve.

ABOVE **Add a protein like tuna to baked potato to balance the high "GI" level.**

products, especially whole-wheat bread and crispbreads) have a high glycemic index, meaning that they release glucose very quickly into the blood. Examine the Glycemic Index extract on page 134 and ensure that you eat foods in the low to moderate range only, or when eating high GI foods, make sure they are properly balanced with protein, such as baked potato with fish or bean curd and salad, not just a baked potato and salad. If you follow the "thirds" idea below, however, your protein and carbohydrate should always be reasonably balanced.

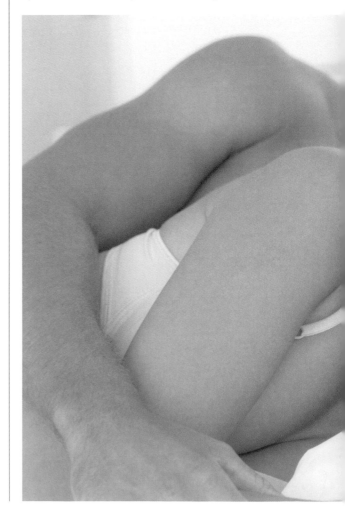

Some foods you may have been eating might be ones that actually make you feel hungry because they raise blood-sugar very quickly. A rise in blood-sugar causes insulin release from the pancreas to deal with this, but sometimes the mechanism overshoots and blood-sugar drops below maintenance level. Two things happen—you feel hungry or you feel tired (or both). Unfortunately, this occurs a lot in those individuals who have eaten a typical Western diet for a long time, especially where the emphasis has been placed on high carbohydrate foods (and especially where these are refined and processed breads, and pastas). There is a lot of evidence to show that even some healthy typical dieters foods (baked potato, wheat

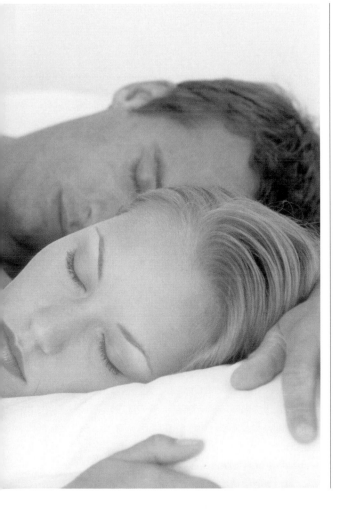

RIGHT Divide your plate into three and use one third for carbohydrates…

LEFT … one third for proteins…

RIGHT …and a slightly larger third for a good, colorful mix of vegetables.

MACRONUTRIENT BALANCE

Re-read the section on a balanced diet on pages 20–23 to get a better idea of the proportion of carbohydrate, fat, and protein required and begin to balance these foods, by eye, to obviate the necessity for that awful weighing process. Imagine a moderate-sized plate and in your mind's eye divide it into approximate thirds—one third will be lean protein (chicken, turkey, lean meat, oily fish, bean curd, pulses), one third will be a whole-grain carbohydrate (buckwheat, basmati brown rice, quinoa, millet, polenta, or even a little whole-wheat pasta), and the remaining third (make this third a little larger!) a good color mix of fresh vegetables or salad vegetables. Use a small amount of good quality olive oil for a dressing (this will be part of the fat ratio). For a dessert afterward, have some live soy (or goat or sheep) yogurt with some fresh fruit, a few pumpkin seeds, and some ground flaxseeds—this gives you protein from the yogurt and seeds, carbohydrate from the fruit and seeds, and essential fatty acids ("good" fat) from the seeds. Eating in this way will also provide a good fiber intake, masses of minerals and vitamins, and other essential nutrients, such as the fatty acids already mentioned. Once the body begins to receive all the micronutrients it needs, metabolism will be enhanced. Drink lots of filtered or bottled water and cut down on stimulants like tea and coffee—these will only disturb your blood-sugar levels and make you feel hungry sooner. Exercise also improves blood-sugar balance within the body.

LEFT Be sure to get plenty of rest—it will improve your general sense of well-being.

IMPROVE YOUR BRAIN POWER AND MEMORY

BELOW Take regular brisk walks in the fresh air to supply the blood with pollutant-free oxygen

Many factors can affect brain power—stress, illness, aging, tobacco, prescribed and recreational drugs, toxin build-up, alcohol, lack of oxygen, and lack of nutrients. Fortunately, there is much you can do to enhance memory and boost mental agility through lifestyle and nutritional changes.

The brain is the control area of the body; it makes up the central nervous system (CNS) together with the spinal cord. The CNS is intricately connected to the peripheral nervous system, which comprises all the nerve fibers (neurones) throughout the body. External stimuli are received by sense organs, converted into electrical messages and sent via sensory neurones to the brain to produce sensations of sight, smell, taste, hearing, balance, pressure, touch, and pain. The brain also receives information from internal organs with regard to its position in space, posture, the contractile state of its various muscles, and the levels of many substances which may need regulating (for example, carbon dioxide and glucose in the blood). Of much of this "input" we are totally unaware. More obvious are the decisions we make, the thoughts we have, the things we remember, the actions we order our body to carry out, the feelings we have, the learning to which we—all of these actions, thoughts, and feelings constitute "output." It is this that is generally regarded as the "brain power" we are seeking to improve.

BELOW Optimal dietary levels of vitamins and minerals are likely to improve brain function.

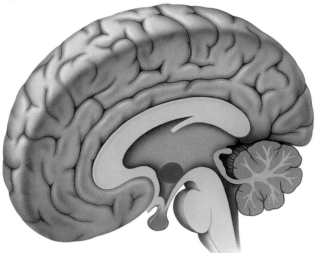

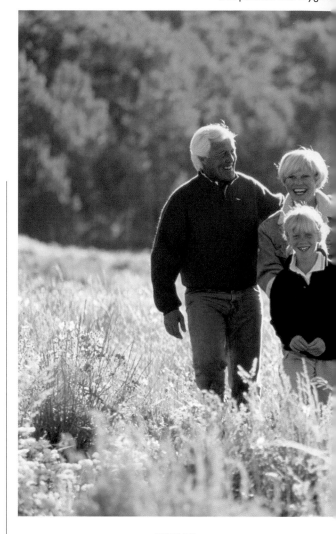

STRESS

A major symptom of stress and aging is reduced mental performance. Recent research has shown that extreme stress can significantly impair memory in as little as four days. Psychologists have known for some time that prolonged stress can cause amnesia and other memory defects; many experts suspect that the hormone cortisol (produced by the adrenals) is involved, since this becomes very active in the brain when people are stressed. Proper nourishment of the adrenals, by eating foods high in the B vitamins (especially B5), will help regulate production of this hormone. The B-complex of vitamins (especially B1, B3, B12, choline, and inositol), and manganese, are important for other aspects of brain function, since they are all needed for effective nerve function. Research has demonstrated that deficiencies of folic acid and other B vitamins can lead to memory loss, mental confusion, depression, and cognitive impairment.

Replace aluminum cookware with stainless steel or glass, exchange your toothpaste and antiperspirant for a natural formulation, do not use cooking foil, and check all medicines for aluminum. Other sources of aluminum include cake mixes, drinking water, flour, pickles, and processed cheese so these need to be avoided too. The only way to ensure that you eliminate as much heavy metal toxicity (and other toxins) in your food and water, is to consume organic produce and filter your tap water. By removing many of these toxins, we are one step nearer to preventing conditions like Parkinson's disease and Alzheimer's disease.

ALCOHOL

Overuse of alcohol can directly damage cells in the brain and nervous system, leaving fewer and fewer cells for all its many functions. Much of this damage is caused by free radicals. Many people enjoy a glass of wine with their meals and, indeed, red wine in moderation contains many antioxidants that can deactivate free radicals and help improve blood flow to the brain. Antioxidant nutrients such as zinc are also important. If alcohol is restricted to one or two glasses of wine three or four times a week and is not taken on an empty stomach, there should be no harm caused.

EXERCISE

We all know that if the brain is deprived of oxygen it dies very quickly, but many of us are short-changing our brain tissue by giving it just enough to tick over, but not enough to function at its maximum. Herbs like Ginkgo biloba may assist in improving peripheral blood flow, especially to the brain. However, regular, gentle, aerobic exercise, like brisk walking, is the best way to fully oxygenate the blood so that the brain receives as much as it needs. But take your exercise as far away from roads and other pollution-generating areas as possible; you don't want to take in toxins with your oxygen. Deep breathing at various points in the day will also refresh the brain by giving it a little bit of extra oxygen.

BELOW Eat foods high in B-complex vitamins to maintain healthy brain function.

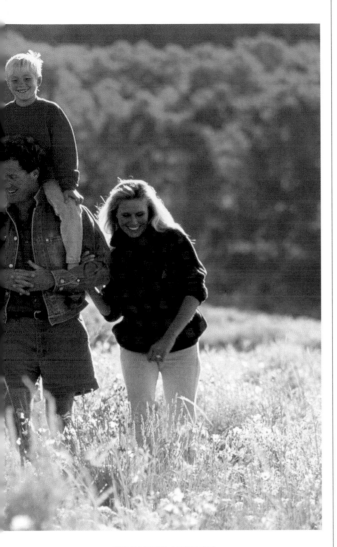

HEALTHY NERVES

Nerve fibers also require the minerals sodium, potassium, calcium, and magnesium to function properly in the conduction of nervous impulses. If any of these minerals is deficient, or if their correct balance is disturbed, there will be inappropriate conduction or interruption in the flow of impulses. Pollutants, such as drugs (prescribed or recreational) and heavy metals (lead, mercury, cadmium, and aluminum) can interfere with the intricate electrical pathways. We need to eliminate as many of these pollutants as possible from our immediate environment, and especially from our diet. However, you must never stop taking prescribed medication, without first discussing this with your physician. Lead may be found in pollutant gases, cadmium is found in tobacco smoke, and aluminum is ubiquitous—cookware, toothpaste, antiperspirants, indigestion remedies, aspirin, and cooking foil have all been found to contain it.

ginger

bean sprouts

mussels

sardines

blackcurra

carrot

apple

lean meat

oats, barley,
and brown rice

oyster

hazelnuts

BRAIN FOOD

For the brain and nervous system to work correctly, many different substances are required. One of the main neurotransmitters contains choline, which is found in lecithin (soy, eggs). Other neurotransmitter chemicals are made from protein, so good-quality proteins need to be supplied—fish, lean meat, bean curd, pulses, and nuts and seeds.

Vitamin C, from fruit and vegetables, and other nutrients are needed for the production of neurotransmitters and protection against free-radical damage. If too much or too little neurotransmitter is produced, this may lead to depression. The minerals needed for nerve function have been listed above, but nerve fibers also need to be insulated correctly. For this, we need a good frequent supply of essential fatty acids; the brain itself is made up of over 50 percent of these. Reduction in the insulation layer causes nerves to misfire or to fail in transmitting impulses. These effects can be seen in diseases like multiple sclerosis.

To help reform nervous insulation, the diet needs to be low in saturated fats and high in essential fatty acids, found in foods like oily fish, pumpkin seeds, flaxseeds and many other natural foods—nuts, pulses, fruits, and all kinds of other vegetables.

basil

rosemary

celery

ABOVE You are what your eat, as this face of food suggests! A sensible diet containing plenty of wholegrains, fresh fish and meat, and fresh vegetables and fruit will help you maintain a healthy body and an alert mind.

STEPS TO IMPROVE BRAIN FUNCTION

• Eat plenty of fresh, organic vegetables, fruit, whole grains, seeds, nuts, and pulses.

• Avoid all refined and processed foods.

• Take some soy lecithin granules and wheat-germ with your cereals for extra nutrients.

• Ensure a good supply of oxygen to the brain with deep breathing and frequent, gentle, aerobic exercise.

• Make lifestyle changes to avoid as much stress as possible.

• Ensure you have adequate sleep and frequent periods of proper relaxation.

• Avoid as many pollutants as possible, especially exhaust gases, tobacco smoke, paints, aerosols, heavy metals like aluminum, and toxins in food and water (including pesticides).

• Carry out detoxification periodically throughout the year; there are many versions of detoxification diets, but ones based on brown rice, vegetables, fruits, and seeds with a little fish are more filling.

• Drink alcohol in moderation, with food if possible; red wine is probably the best.

• Drink plenty of bottled or filtered water daily.

• Take a daily multiformula supplement; make sure it contains good levels of all the B vitamins (especially B12, folic acid, choline, and inositol); antioxidant nutrients (vitamins A, C, and E, and the minerals zinc and selenium); minerals (calcium, magnesium, manganese, and potassium); and fish oils or flaxseed oil.

BRAIN ENERGY

Brain activity requires a continuous supply of energy; this it must obtain from glucose in the blood supply. One of the reasons for poor concentration and dizziness is lack of energy in the brain. However, giving the brain a "quick-fix" from sugary food is not the answer, because of the rebound effect of insulin. What is required is food which will supply glucose in a slow-release, constant way. Food with a low to moderate glycemic index (GI) such as whole grains (particularly rye, oats, and brown basmati rice), and pulses are the best. Refer to the Glycemic Index section on page 134.

ABOVE **They may be tempting, but "quick-fix" foods are best taken only as a rare treat.**

LEFT **Eating foods rich in vitamin C can improve the production of neurotransmitters in the brain; this can help with depression.**

DEAL WITH STRESS

Stress is a major factor in disease. It comes from a variety of sources, some of which are familiar—time constraints, relationships, family, emotions, job and money pressures. Environmental pressures also stress the body—pollution, noise, housing problems, cold, or overheating. In addition to this, a high intake of toxins, or a nutrient-poor diet high in processed, refined, and "chemical" food will add chemical stresses of which we are not totally aware.

ABOVE Eat plenty of fresh, vitamin-C-packed fruit to help you deal with stress more easily.

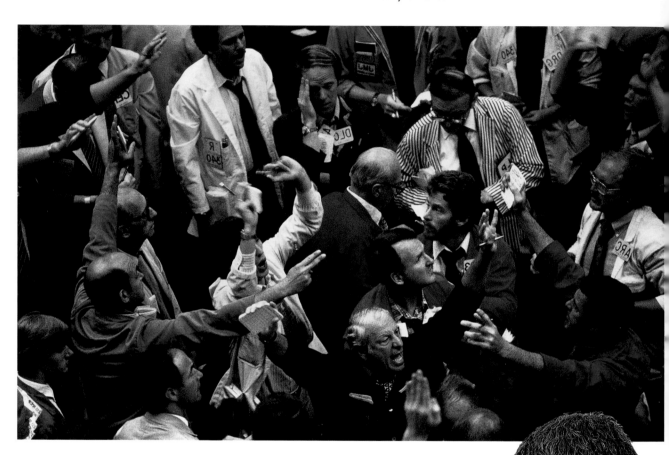

Our ability to deal with stress is under the control of the endocrine (hormonal) system. Stress induces a series of reactions known as the "fight or flight" mechanism, when the body acts in a coordinated fashion to prepare itself for physical action and energy expenditure.

The first, immediate effect is caused by the brain stimulating the adrenal glands to secrete the hormone adrenaline. Adrenaline acts on the liver, encouraging it to convert stored glycogen to glucose, which it releases into the bloodstream. Blood pressure and heart rate increase to let this "emergency" glucose be conveyed to the muscles where it will be needed for movement. Breathing rate is also increased to bring the oxygen to the cells for energy release. Digestion stops as blood is diverted to the muscles to prepare them for action, and blood platelets get ready to aggregate should they need to form a blood

ABOVE Most jobs are stressful to some degree—these dealers on the Chicago Stock Exchange are an extreme example. The body reacts to stressful situations by producing hormones that are helpful in the short term, but can produce problems over a long period of time.

RIGHT Stressful situations occur throughout our daily lives, and these can affect our general well-being.

LEFT To help counteract the effects of stress, you should take frequent short breaks and do some deep breathing; a yoga class may be particularly effective.

STEPS FOR DEALING WITH STRESS

• Eat a nutrient-dense wholefood diet; whole grains, pulses, seeds, nuts, oily fish, lean meat, live yogurt, and masses of a good color mix of fresh vegetables and fruit.

• Add wheat germ and ground flaxseeds to your cereals for extra B vitamins.

• Avoid all processed and refined foods (especially sugary foods, which are most attractive when we feel stressed).

• Enjoy a little good wine with a meal, but try not to use alcohol as a stress-reliever.

• Vitamin C is great for helping in times of stress; have plenty of high vitamin C fruits and vegetables like kiwi fruit, guavas, blackcurrants, and tomato, and/or take a vitamin C supplement of around 500mg two or three times a day.

• Try some herbal infusions and teas instead of stimulants like tea, coffee, and cola drinks: lemon balm, camomile, verbena, passiflora, and lavender—all of these are excellent for encouraging calm and relaxation.

• Extracts of blue–green algae (spirulina and chlorella) act as antioxidants and are a good all-round supplemental source of naturally balanced vitamins, minerals, enzymes, and amino acids—or take a daily multiformula that has high levels of B vitamins (especially B1, B2, B5, and B6), vitamin E, magnesium, and boron.

• Avoid tobacco smoke, and as many environmental toxins as possible; for example, avoid pesticides in food by eating organic produce.

• Embark on a detoxification diet at an appropriate time.

• Gently exercise as often as you can; oxygenate the system.

• Take frequent short breaks to stretch muscles and do some deep breathing, or take a yoga class.

• Try an aromatherapy massage or meditate; both excellent ways to relax.

clot over any wound that may occur. In addition, stress stimulates the pituitary gland to produce hormones that act on the adrenals to release a group of hormones called the corticoids. These further help in making glucose available for energy, and in the retention of sodium for increased nervous transmission.

It is easy to see how this orchestrated process enables the human body to deal with dangerous situations, but in modern humans, these physiological reactions to stress remain, while the triggers and the effects are completely different. The cumulative effects of raised blood glucose, increased blood pressure, enhanced heart and breathing rates, and increased blood clotting, is our body's "adaptive response" to deal with threatening or demanding situations. But when this occurs over and over again with very little activity actually taking place, it is obviously going to cause problems. Stress is not, then, an illness in itself, but rather a response by the body to anything that puts a strain upon it. Illnesses resulting from, or exacerbated by, stress can include high blood pressure, heart disease, arthritis, asthma, insomnia, anorexia, obesity, and eczema.

Hormonal imbalance and metabolic exhaustion are the casualties of an overstressed lifestyle. Fortunately, there is a lot we can do to nourish the exhausted glands and rebalance our metabolism.

RIGHT **Packed with vitamin C, tomatoes are a great stress-buster.**

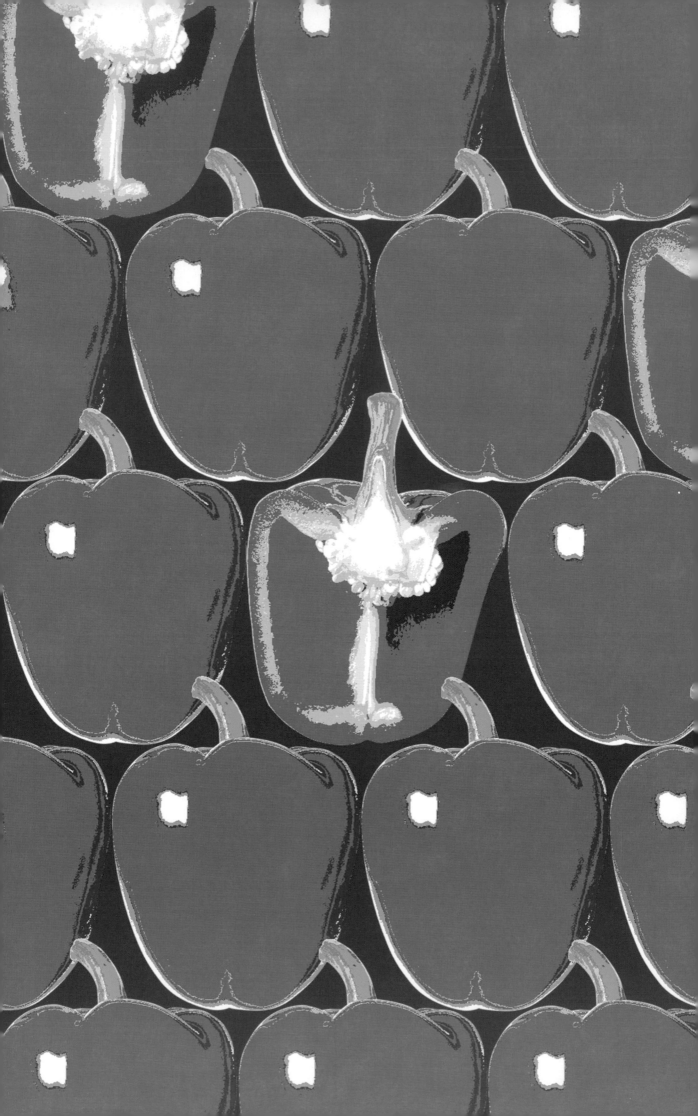

PART FIVE

PROBLEM SOLVING

Vitamins and minerals can be beneficial in the treatment of virtually all chronic diseases, even those for which no effective drugs are yet known. In fact, vitamins in sufficient doses, taken under the supervision of trained nutritionists or dieticians, can help you to cut down or eliminate some of the drugs you may be taking. However, as with all things, do exercise caution, and do not ever consider giving up necessary medication in favor of supplements without the supervision of your physician and a trained, registered therapist. Don't try to take every piece of advice given here for your condition: pick and choose among the suggestions for the nutritional supplement you believe will suit you and your lifestyle.

THE SKIN, HAIR, AND NAILS

The skin is the largest organ we have. It is a "barometer" of our state of health and any poor lifestyle or nutritional habits will affect its appearance. A stressful lifestyle, lack of sleep, and a diet low in the essential vitamins and minerals will eventually show up in the complexion. Recently, greater emphasis has been placed on treating skin problems from the inside (by good nutrition) rather than by the use of creams and lotions from the outside. A lifestyle that reduces the level of free radicals, together with a good basic diet of wholefoods and antioxidant-rich vegetables and fruit, will prevent and heal some of the damage.

ABOVE **A good intake of nutrients will result in strong, healthy nails.**

The lower layers of the skin are made up of living cells. Changes in nutrient levels will affect these cells to varying degrees, resulting in dryness, soreness, rash, pimples, and other irritating skin conditions.

The most common environmental agents affecting skin integrity are the free radicals that attack it, both externally from temperature changes, cigarette smoke, pollution, and ultraviolet light, and internally from a diet low in essential nutrients and high in hydrogenated fats and highly processed foods. Free radicals cause cross-linkage between collagen fibers in the skin and encourage wrinkle formation as elasticity decreases.

The antioxidant vitamin C is of particular importance in maintaining a youthful skin, since it is an essential nutrient for the formation and maintenance of collagen; zinc, boron, silicon, and iodine are also involved in collagen formation.

Anthocyanidins—a group of phytochemicals that are to be found in blue/purple fruits—have become the main focus of researchers' attention, alongside investigation into the nutrients that are involved in collagen maintenance.

Since hair is a product of the skin, poor hair condition and scalp disorders will be a direct cause of problems with the skin. Healthy hair is dependent upon good blood circulation carrying adequate levels of essential nutrients (especially vitamins B2, B3, B5, folic acid, biotin, choline, and inositol, and selenium and manganese). For appropriate pigment production of skin and hair, copper and manganese are required. Problems related to poor blood circulation will adversely affect the structure of the nails, since these too are a product of the skin. If the scalp or nail bed are not nourished properly, fungal and bacterial diseases can take hold. Acute periods of illness will often be evident in the nails, where bumps and striations, grooves or streaks indicate a period of poor nutrient supply to the nail bed. However, during a fever, hair and nails may grow faster as the rise in temperature increases the rate of metabolism. Low levels of minerals, especially iron, may produce "spoon-shaped" nails.

BELOW **A range of vitamins and nutrients are essential for healthy hair.**

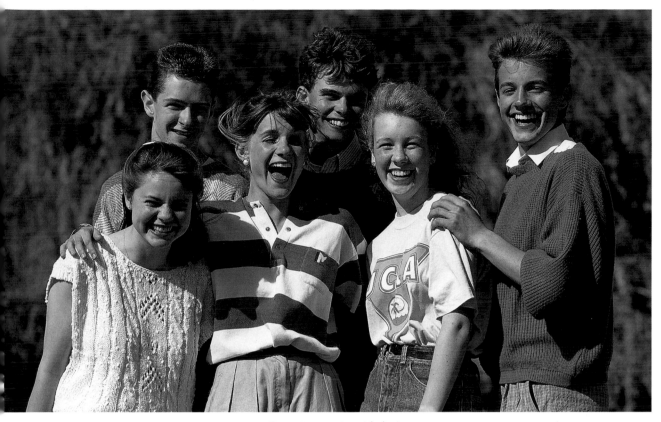

ABOVE Continuing a nutrient-rich diet into
adolescence is vital for avoiding acne.

ACNE

Acne is caused by the over-production of an oily substance called sebum. The pores become blocked and spots and pimples are the result. Acne is very common among adolescents because of hormonal changes affecting the production rate of sebum.

Acne can be the result of: poor gut flora, a sluggish liver, hormones and the contraceptive pill, excess intake of saturated fats and refined carbohydrates, low fiber, dairy foods, food intolerance, and nutrient deficiency (in vitamins A, B6, folic acid, C, and E, essential fatty acids, zinc, and chromium).

COLD SORES

Cold sores are caused by the herpes simplex virus. They generally occur around the mouth and are very contagious; care should be taken not to spread them to other parts of the body or to other people. The virus can lie dormant in the body and only flare up when the immune system is underfunctioning.

Cold sores can be precipitated premenstrually and by: stress, fatigue, sub-optimum nutrition, foods high in the amino acid argenine (peanuts, bean curd, soybeans, gelatin, chocolate, carob, coconut, oats, whole wheat, and wheatgerm), infections, and illness.

NUTRITIONAL HELP FOR ACNE

- Live yogurt (to replenish healthy gut flora)—can also be applied directly to the skin.

- Soluble fibers and pectins, from oats, fruits, and vegetables—reduce intake of wheat.

- Mixed freshly ground seeds—sesame, pumpkin, sunflower, and flaxseeds.

- Plenty of vegetables and fruit, particularly those containing the antioxidants (vitamins A, C, E and the minerals selenium and zinc).

- Supplements: B-complex and extra B6; zinc; antioxidant formula (vitamin A, C, E, and selenium); chromium; fish oils.

NUTRITIONAL HELP FOR COLD SORES

- Vitamin C-rich fruit and vegetables (to boost immune function).

- Garlic (as an antiviral, and to boost immune function).

- Zinc-rich foods—fish, pumpkin seeds, ginger root, pecans.

- lysine-rich foods—fish, chicken, beef, lamb, milk, cheese, beans, Brewer's yeast, and mung bean sprouts.

- Plenty of fruit and vegetables (for immune-boosting micronutrients in general).

- Supplements: a good multiformula (containing zinc), vitamins C and E; *Acidophilus*; garlic perles; l-lysine.

ECZEMA

Eczema is an itchy, inflamed skin condition wherein the skin becomes red and flaky and may also have tiny blisters leading to weepy sores and scabs, making it open to secondary bacterial infection. Eczema can be a result of: sensitivity to detergents (contact eczema or allergy, an inherited condition, associated with other allergies like hayfever and asthma), food intolerance (cow's milk, egg, wheat, red meat, sugar, tea, coffee, alcohol), stress, low stomach acid, sluggish liver, saturated or hydrogenated fats, food additives, chlorinated water, and nutrient deficiencies (especially essential fatty acids and zinc).

NUTRITIONAL HELP FOR ECZEMA

- A good wholefood diet
- A daily serving of freshly ground seeds, especially pumpkin and flaxseed.
- A small amount of either diluted freshly squeezed lemon or diluted cider vinegar with the main meal of the day (to improve stomach acidity).
- Plenty of filtered or bottled water between meals.

- Anthocyanidin-containing fruits—blueberries, cherries, blackcurrants.
- Bean curd, pulses, and a little oily fish as main proteins.
- Supplements: Vitamins A, B-complex (including biotin, choline, and inositol), C, and E; zinc; fish oils; evening primrose oil; vitamin E applied directly to the skin to prevent scarring and improve flexibility.

PSORIASIS

Psoriasis is a noncontagious skin condition that commonly affects the knees, elbows, shins, below the breasts, and scalp; it can, however, affect any part of the skin. It appears on the skin as bright pink, raised patches with white scales, although other types display characteristics such as pus-like blisters or severe sloughing of the skin. Its main cause is overproduction of epidermal cells. This can be triggered by several factors, including the following: heavy alcohol consumption, stress, low-nutrient diet (especially essential fatty acids), nutritional deficiencies (antioxidants, folic acid and other B vitamins, selenium, zinc), low intake of fiber, excess meat, excess refined food and saturated fat, food intolerance (citrus fruits, tomatoes), poor acid/alkaline balance, and sluggish liver.

NUTRITIONAL HELP FOR PSORIASIS

- A daily serving of freshly ground mixed seeds, especially pumpkin seeds.
- A daily serving of freshly ground mixed seeds, especially pumpkin seeds.
- Plenty of fruits and vegetables (for their alkaline-forming activity)—except citrus fruits and tomatoes.
- High fiber/high pectin fruits and vegetables—string beans, carrots, apples.
- Brown rice, millet, buckwheat, and quinoa as main whole grains; avoid wheat, oats, barley, and rye.
- Plenty of filtered or bottled water between meals.
- Supplements: fish oils; a good multiformula (including good levels of zinc and selenium, and vitamins

D and E); Milk thistle herb (to improve liver detoxification); lipase (to help digest fats).Plenty of fruits and vegetables (for their alkaline-forming activity)—except citrus fruits and tomatoes.
- High fiber/high pectin fruits and vegetables—string beans, carrots, apples.
- Brown rice, millet, buckwheat, and quinoa as main whole grains; avoid wheat, oats, barley, and rye.
- Plenty of filtered or bottled water between meals.
- Supplements: fish oils; a good multiformula (including good levels of zinc and selenium, and vitamins D and E); Milk thistle herb (to improve liver detoxification); lipase (to help digest fats).

RIGHT **A good wholefood diet will help with the symptoms of eczema or psoriasis.**

GENERAL HAIR LOSS AND ALOPECIA

Hair loss can be a mild condition in which there is sporadic loss from the head as well as all over the body. This can sometimes occur during pregnancy. On the other hand, it may be a severe condition where most of the hair is lost, although this sometimes occurs at one spot on the scalp only. Hair loss can be caused by: poor nourishment of the hormonal system (especially the thyroid, adrenals, and pituitary); nutrient deficiency (vitamin B6, biotin, folic acid, inositol); excess refined food and sugar, excess alcohol, nicotine, heavy metal toxicity, low level of antioxidants, and crash dieting.

NUTRITIONAL HELP FOR ALOPECIA

• Plenty of vegetables and fruit (for antioxidants and micronutrients).

• Lightly cooked or steamed fibrous vegetables like carrots and green beans.

• A daily serving of freshly ground mixed seeds (to help hormonal function).

• Wheat germ added to cereals, soups, stews, and yogurt (extra B vitamins).

• Oily fish and lean meat, and pulses for protein.

• Soy milk and bean curd (for phyto-estrogens).

• Supplements: a good multiformula (including high levels of beta-carotene, B-complex with folic acid and biotin, vitamins C and E, iron, zinc, selenium, iodine); lecithin; fish oils; evening primrose oil.

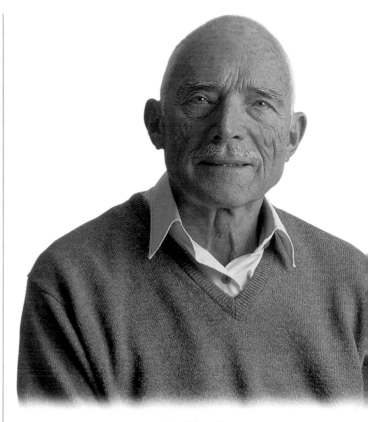

ABOVE **A good multiformula supplement may help slow hair loss.**

DANDRUFF

Dandruff is flaking of the scalp and is usually associated with a yeast infection; bacterial infections can also occur. Dandruff is caused, or exacerbated by: an acid-forming diet, excess carbohydrates and sugar, excess saturated and hydrogenated fats, excess alcohol, excess salt, excess citrus fruit, poor antioxidant intake, food intolerance (wheat, dairy, and other common allergens), poor intake of essential fatty acids and high vitamin B foods, and poor digestive activity.

NUTRITIONAL HELP FOR DANDRUFF

• Plenty of dark green and orange vegetables and fruits, except citrus.

• A daily serving of freshly ground mixed seeds (especially pumpkin seeds), nuts, oatgerm/oatmeal, and avocados.

• Some raw vegetables and sprouted seeds every day (to improve enzyme levels).

• Fish, shellfish, and pulses.

• Brown rice, millet, buckwheat, and quinoa as main carbohydrates, but reduce levels of carbohydrates in general.

• Supplements: vitamin A or beta-carotene; vitamin B-complex (especially B6, B12, and folic acid); selenium; zinc; evening primrose oil; lecithin; digestive enzymes.

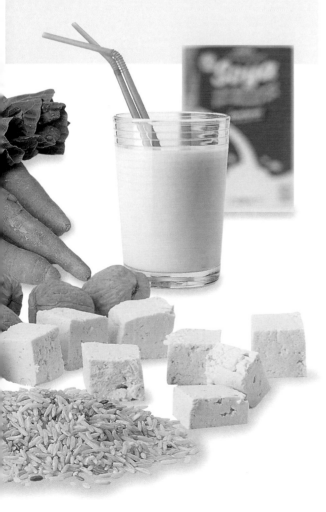

157

THE RESPIRATORY SYSTEM

BELOW An allergy to ci[?] may cause respiratory problems.

We can live without food or water for weeks and days respectively, but without air we can survive only a few minutes. Any disease, microbial infection, or allergic reactions which restrict the intake of air, seriously affect general health since they impede the proper flow of oxygen and prevent the production of energy in the tissues. Fortunately, there are nutrients that can protect the lungs from damage and disease.

The respiratory organs—lungs, respiratory muscles, diaphragm—provide a set of "bellows" to bring oxygen into close contact with the bloodstream. The interface of lung lining and blood is made up of thin, moist, delicate membranes which enable maximum exchange of respiratory gases—oxygen in, carbon dioxide out—on a regular basis.

Many of the nutrients essential for a healthy respiratory system are antioxidants which neutralize free radicals and boost the immune system. In addition, keeping mucous-generating foods (dairy and refined carbohydrates) and common allergens (wheat, citrus, egg) low will help keep the airways open.

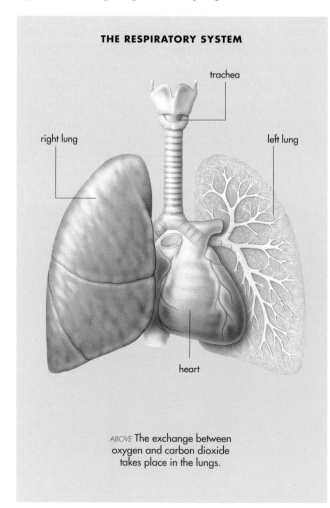

THE RESPIRATORY SYSTEM

trachea

right lung

left lung

heart

ABOVE The exchange between oxygen and carbon dioxide takes place in the lungs.

NUTRITIONAL HELP FOR ASTHMA

- Plenty of vegetables and fruits (except citrus), especially those high in antioxidants.

- Blue/purple fruits, for their anthocyanidins.

- High-magnesium foods such as dark green vegetables, nuts, and seeds.

- High-selenium foods such as Brazil nuts, oats, and garlic (be careful with garlic if you are sensitive to sulfur in foods).

- Have some seeds every days, especially pumpkin seeds (for their immune-boosting zinc content) and ground flaxseeds (for their essential fatty acids and as an alternative to fish).

- Eat onions frequently— they have antiasthmatic properties.

- For your protein, eat foods from a vegetable source (bean curd and beans).

- Sip a little diluted cider vinegar with your main meal to help improve stomach acidity.

- Drink plenty of diluted fruit juices and bottled/filtered water between meals.

- Supplements: a high dose multivitamin formula with vitamins A, B5, B6, B12 and folic acid; an antioxidant formula; a multimineral with magnesium and calcium in a 2:1 ratio, zinc, molybdenum, silica, and selenium.

ASTHMA

Its main symptoms are wheeziness, breathlessness, and chest tightness. Allergens such as dust, animal fur, and pollen can trigger an attack, as can infections, tobacco smoke, anxiety, stress, or overstrenuous exercise. The main dietary causes include: excess salt (increases sensitivity to histamine); sulfite sensitivity (sulfured fruits); food intolerance (wheat, refined carbohydrates, dairy foods, sugar, food additives, tap water, some meats, some fish, eggs, coffee, tea, and chocolate); insufficient stomach acid; nutrient deficiencies (vitamins A, B6, B12, and C, magnesium, selenium).

COLDS AND FLU

One hundred different, but related, viruses cause colds. Symptoms include a runny sore nose, sneezing, coughing, and a sore throat. Influenza is also caused by several related viruses and its symptoms are similar but more severe—fever, aching muscles, sore throat, headache, and weakness. In the cold and flu season, you need to increase those foods which help to boost the immune system. If you feel a cold or flu starting, take immediate action as follows:

• Drink plenty of bottled or filtered water.

• Drink hot lemon made with freshly-sliced lemons (include rind and pith), honey, and vitamin C powder—alternatively, drink diluted elderberry extract.

• If you can't face food, just have a little thin soup made from chicken bouillon, crushed garlic, and vegetable juice.

• Eat an onion baked with a little brown sugar (good for sore throats and coughs).

• Supplements: Vitamin C (best as a powder added to hot lemon), 1,000mg every two or three hours; zinc lozenges; Echinacea; vitamin A drops (add to hot lemon if required).

BRONCHITIS

Inflammatory reactions occur in the mucous lining of the air passages causing bronchitis and resulting in "productive" coughing, breathlessness, wheeziness, and chest pains. Acute attacks are caused by infections and are short-lived. The main dietary causes include: excess carbohydrates and dairy foods; acid-forming foods; toxicity; food intolerances (animal products, refined carbohydrates, sugar, alcohol, wheat); nutrient deficiencies (vitamins A, B-complex, C, and E, zinc).

NUTRITIONAL HELP FOR BRONCHITIS

• Plenty of dark green and orange vegetables and fruits.

• Eat buckwheat, millet, brown rice, and quinoa as main carbohydrates.

• Eat pulses for protein, where meat and fish sensitivity occurs.

• Have a daily serving of freshly ground mixed seeds, especially pumpkin seeds (to boost the immune system).

• Supplements: Vitamin C (1,000mg twice a day for a month or so); antioxidant formula with selenium and zinc; B-complex.

HAYFEVER

Hayfever, or allergic rhinitis, is caused by an allergy to one or several types of pollen. It produces irritation of the mucous membranes lining the nose and throat, which leads to a runny nose and red, itchy, runny eyes, and can be made worse by stress, excess carbohydrate, and food intolerances (wheat, refined carbohydrates, sugar, cow's milk and other dairy foods, coffee, tea, alcohol, soft drinks, and some meats).

NUTRITIONAL HELP FOR HAYFEVER

• Plenty of all types of vegetables and fruits, except citrus and any others that produce allergic reactions.

• Millet, buckwheat, brown rice, and quinoa as main carbohydrates; avoid refined carbohydrates; and reduce total carbohydrate intake .

• A daily serving of freshly ground mixed seeds (especially pumpkin seeds) and nuts.

• Supplements: an antioxidant formula; a high-potency B-complex with B5 and B6; vitamin C with bioflavonoids; digestive enzymes containing proteases; zinc; bee pollen supplement.

LEFT Both asthma and bronchitis result in wheeziness and breathlessness.

THE IMMUNE SYSTEM

The immune system protects us against infectious diseases and also against errors in cell division that may result in cancers and tumors. There are many different types of microorganism (viruses, bacteria, yeasts, molds, protozoal parasites) that have the power to do us a great deal of harm if our immune function is poor.

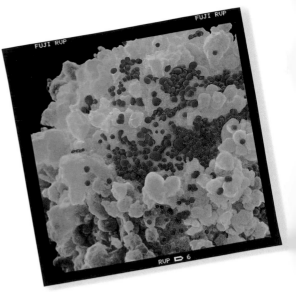

ABOVE The HIV virus that causes AIDS is shown here in red on the surface of a human white blood cell.

Our first line of defense is to prevent entry of microbes into the body by maintaining healthy skin, mucous membranes, and stomach acid.

The second is to disarm those agents that do enter. It is the second of these two mechanisms that is popularly referred to as the immune system, the main army of which is composed of various types of white cell that attack the invader in many different ways, including the production of antibodies and neutralization of microbial toxins. A whole host of nutrients are involved in keeping the immune system at the peak of function, and a good-quality, wholefood diet with plenty of fresh vegetables is extremely helpful in this regard. Additionally, when infections do strike, taking immune-boosting supplements, like vitamins A and C and zinc, can make an enormous difference to the speed of the healing process.

The formation of cancers and tumors tends to be a lengthier process involving not only poor nutrient levels, but also substances called carcinogens. Common carcinogens include tobacco smoke, barbecued and smoked foods, nitrosamines, free radicals, pollutants, environmental estrogens, insecticides, pesticides, and radiation. When body tissues have to deal with an excessive carcinogenic load, especially if nutrient intake is poor, cell division cannot be properly controlled. If this is not detected by roving members of the immune army, then this rapidly dividing group of cells becomes a growth. Therefore, it is vital to avoid as many carcinogens as possible by eating good wholesome food devoid of additives, pesticides, and other substances, and to make lifestyle changes such as giving up smoking. Recent research indicates that many cancers (well over one third) could be prevented, and some even treated, by proper nutrition and improved lifestyles.

FACTORS THAT WEAKEN THE IMMUNE SYSTEM

- Surgery.
- Antibiotics and other drugs.
- Some digestive disorders (enzyme deficiencies, low stomach acid, chronic constipation).
- Candida infections.
- Poor nutrient intake.
- Pollution.
- Stress.
- Genetic predisposition.
- Colds and flu—see page 159.

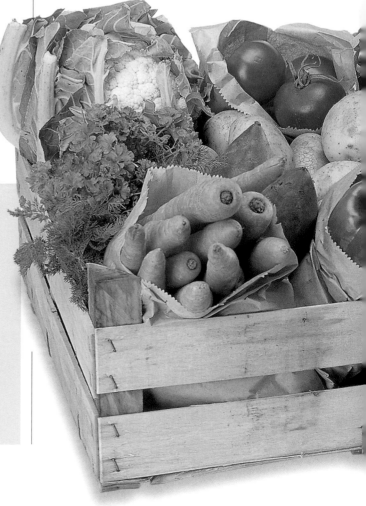

AIDS AND HIV

The human immunodeficiency virus (HIV) remains in the body for life once infection has taken place through direct contact with infected body fluids (blood, semen, vaginal fluids, breastmilk). However, if steps are taken to improve lifestyle and maximize intake of essential nutrients, the virus can remain dormant for periods of several years. Unfortunately, in certain circumstances, the virus enters its lytic cycle and the disease becomes acquired immune deficiency syndrome (AIDS), where the T-helper cells of the immune system are rapidly destroyed.

Most of the symptoms of AIDS are related to impaired immunity, which can lead to the appearance of vigorous opportunistic infections and skin cancers. Both HIV and AIDS respond well to nutritional therapy and suitable supplementation.

GENERALIZED POOR IMMUNE FUNCTION

Since infection of any type (colds, catarrh, coughs, sore throats, influenza; and areas where wounds and burns are slow to heal) concerns the activity of microorganisms, anything that reduces immune function (low levels of vitamins A and C, zinc, bioflavonoids, antioxidants) will automatically give these organisms opportunity. A high toxic load and overuse of alcohol will also interfere with the efficacy of the immune system.

NUTRITIONAL HELP FOR AIDS AND HIV

- Plenty of dark green and orange vegetables and fruit (for their antioxidant activity and their alkalizing effect).

- Garlic taken daily (for its antimicrobial properties and its germanium content).

- Shiitake mushrooms (for their immune-boosting properties).

- A daily serving of freshly ground mixed seeds, especially pumpkin seeds and flaxseeds.

- Raw vegetables, and sprouted seeds and pulses daily (for their natural enzyme content to help proper digestion).

- Unpolluted oily fish, bean curd, lean meat, live soy yogurt for protein; avoid dairy food.

- Whole grains (brown rice, millet, quinoa, buckwheat, oats, barley, corn, rye); avoid refined carbohydrates and sugar (to prevent proliferation of yeasts and moulds).

- Avoid saturated fat, hydrogenated fats, alcohol, and common food allergens (wheat, etc.).

- Supplements: a high strength antioxidant formula (vitamins A, C, and E, zinc, selenium); extra vitamin C; a high strength B complex (especially B12); evening primrose oil, fish oil and/or flaxseed oil; lecithin; garlic perles.

NUTRITIONAL HELP FOR POOR IMMUNE FUNCTION

- Maximum intake of vegetables and fruit high in vitamin A (carrots, sweet potato, melons, apricots, mango, peaches, dark green leafy vegetables, and vitamin C (blackcurrants, guava, citrus—this will automatically improve antioxidant levels.

- Garlic and onion, daily if possible.

- A daily serving of freshly ground mixed seeds, especially pumpkin seeds.

- Elderberry cordial or diluted elderberry tincture.

- Minimum grain carbohydrates; obtain carbohydrates mainly from vegetables and fruits.

- Avoid alcohol, nonorganic produce, candy, tea, coffee, milk, and cheese.

- Supplements: vitamins A, C, and E; zinc (zinc and vitamin C lozenges for sore throat); vitamin B-complex (including folic acid); garlic perles; elderberry extract; Echinacea, Golden Seal.

LEFT Immune deficiencies, including those caused by HIV infection and AIDS, respond well to nutritional therapy.

ALLERGIES

The immune system can sometime respond to noninfective and harmless substances. When this happens, the body produces histamine, and an allergic reaction ensues. This can be in the skin, the respiratory system or the digestive tract. Causes of allergies include: genetic factors; food intolerances (wheat, dairy foods, citrus, eggs, nuts); and nutrient deficiencies.

RIGHT A high molybdenum diet can ease the symptoms of thrush and candidiasis.

NUTRITIONAL HELP FOR ALLERGIES

- Eat a good wholefood diet; remove all processed and refined foods.

- Avoid all common allergenic foods including wheat, dairy, citrus, eggs, and any other foods to which you feel you are sensitive.

- Plenty of vegetables, especially garlic, and fruit (except citrus) from the whole color range—orange, red, yellow, green, and purple.

- Drink plenty of bottled or filtered water between meals.

- Eat a mixture of nuts—be aware of nut allergies—and seeds daily (for their essential fatty acids).

- Supplements: a good, well-balanced, multiformula (containing vitamins A, B12, C, and E, and zinc, copper, calcium, magnesium); extra vitamin C and zinc may be needed.

RIGHT **Drinking diluted cranberry juice will help relieve thrush.**

CANDIDIASIS AND THRUSH

Candidiasis and thrush are caused by the yeast *Candida albicans*. Generally yeast infections are called overgrowths, since most people carry low levels. Overgrowths occur when immune function is compromised—excess intake of sugar, hormonal change (pregnancy, contraceptive pill). Many people suffer from a flare-up of *Candida* after taking antibiotics, which kills helpful bacteria and removes microbial competition in the gut. Many women suffer from vaginal thrush, but in some the yeast changes to a mycelial (threadlike) form which penetrates the gut lining. It can then ramify throughout major organs; this is systemic candidiasis, which can also occur in men. Nutritional treatment involves starving the yeast, dealing with yeast "die-off," reinstating helpful bacteria, and preventing nutrient deficiency.

NUTRITIONAL HELP FOR CANDIDIASIS AND THRUSH

- Plenty of fresh vegetables of all types; eat some of these raw.

- Wholegrain carbohydrates except wheat; avoid all refined carbohydrates, honey, sugar, and any other sweet foods.

- Increase your intake of garlic (for its antifungal properties), olive oil, and oily fish.

- Eat high-molybdenum foods—brown rice, pulses, cauliflower, garlic, oats—to detoxify Candida metabolites.

- Plenty of water between meals and diluted cranberry extract (unsweetened variety); Pau d'arco tea is also useful, as is bicarbonate in water.

- For protein, cut down meat and dairy foods and have more vegetable proteins—bean curd, pulses, and seeds and nuts.

- Have live soy yogurt daily.

- Avoid yeast, alcohol, tea, coffee, smoked/pickled meat or fish, and fermented foods.

- Supplements: a multivitamin including A, B complex (especially B6 and biotin), C, and E; zinc; magnesium; high potency garlic; a probiotic (*Lactoacidophilus* and *Bifidus*); fructo-oligosaccharides (to selectively feed the probiotic organisms); cranberry extract.

NUTRITIONAL HELP FOR TUMORS AND CANCERS

- Plenty of raw vegetables and fruits from the whole color range, but especially orange and dark green types (for their antioxidant and potassium content).

- Specific anticancer produce—tomatoes, broccoli, Brussels sprouts, cabbage, hot peppers, onions, garlic, apples, grapes, pink grapefruit, watermelon, guava, raspberries, strawberries, sprouted seeds, shiitake mushrooms, and soy products (soy milk, bean curd, miso) and beans.

- Blue/purple fruits for their anthocyanidins (powerful antioxidants).

- A serving of freshly ground mixed seeds daily.

- Gluten-free grains— brown rice, millet, buckwheat, quinoa (for fiber).

- Oily fish, pulses, soy, and nuts; reduce amount of meat.

- Plenty of bottled or filtered water in between meals.

- Green tea and black tea (reduces incidence of digestive cancers).

- Avoid all saturated and hydrogenated fats, refined and processed food, sugar, smoked/pickled/salt-cured foods, coffee, tea with milk, and alcohol.

- Supplements: natural beta-carotene; B vitamins (especially B6 and folic acid); vitamins C and E; calcium and magnesium; selenium; molybdenum; zinc; fish or flaxseed oil; high potency garlic.

TUMORS AND CANCERS

In a healthy immune system, any abnormal cells should be eradicated. Even where there is genetic predisposition to cancer, a wholesome diet and healthy lifestyle can, in many cases, prevent its onset. Recent research into nutritional control over gene expression ("nutritioneering") is producing some interesting results in the prevention of cancer and other conditions such as heart disease, diabetes, and arthritis. The immune system can, however, be overwhelmed with pollutants and toxins and the "damage limitation" monitoring system may respond poorly at these times. Nutritional causes for the development of cancer include: poor supply of essential nutrients; saturated and hydrogenated fats; low dietary fiber; high processed food; excess alcohol; foods containing nitrosamines (smoked, pickled, and salt-cured foods), "soft" and/or chlorinated water; and food containing toxins, pesticides, and environmental estrogens.

RIGHT Extracts of the Echinacea flower boost the immune system to fight infection.

CHRONIC FATIGUE SYNDROME AND ME (MYALGIC ENCEPHALOMYELITIS)

Chronic fatigue and ME can be seriously debilitating disorders that may last for years. Symptoms include depression, extreme tiredness, muscle fatigue, muscle pains, headaches, memory lapses, and word jumbling. Studies have shown that in some cases, the root cause appears to be due to nerve damage caused by pesticide poisoning (particularly the organophosphates); other studies implicate vaccinations, immune disorders, viral infections, *Candida* overgrowth, stress, high toxicity, food intolerances, poor digestion, and nutrient deficiency.

NUTRITIONAL HELP FOR CHRONIC FATIGUE SYNDROME

- A plentiful intake of antioxidant nutrients from vegetables and fruit

- Lightly steamed vegetables (nutrients more readily available).

- Avoid foods that are difficult to digest—dairy food, some grains and pulses.

- A daily serving of freshly ground mixed seeds, especially pumpkin and flaxseeds.

- Easily digested protein from foods like bean curd, millet, quinoa, "pod" vegetables, seeds, nuts, eggs, and a little oily fish (deep sea—to avoid pollutants).

- Avoid all stimulants (tea, coffee, colds), rich food, common allergenic foods (wheat, dairy, citrus), food additives, processed food, hydrogenated fats, alcohol, non-organic food.

- Supplements: a good multiformula; extra vitamin B12, vitamin C; extra magnesium and zinc; an antioxidant formula; fish oils; evening primrose oil; a probiotic (*Acidophilus* and *Bifidus*); Echinacea, Coenzyme Q10.

- A new supplement, NADH, has been proved successful in many cases.

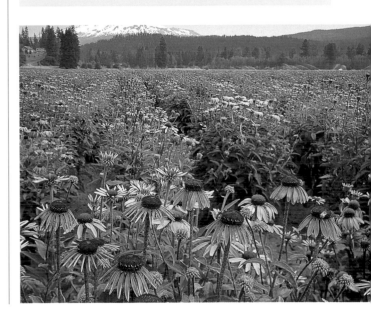

THE URINARY SYSTEM

The urinary system filters and excretes wastes from the bloodstream. This takes place in the many thousands of tiny filtering structures in the kidney called nephrons, from where wastes are transported as urine to the bladder for storage. Urine is released to the outside via a tube called the urethra. This activity is vital to the well-being of the individual, since without it, harmful nitrogenous wastes, like uric acid, will soon build up and prevent normal metabolism from occurring. A diet that is high in animal protein, animal fat, and refined foods puts a great strain on the kidneys. So too will a diet with mineral imbalances and excessive intake of salt.

ABOVE Celery has antidiuretic properties, helpful for flushing the system.

NEPHRITIS, CYSTITIS, AND URETHRITIS

All of these, and associated conditions, relate to inflammation in the various parts of the urinary system. Nephritis is inflammation within the kidneys, cystitis inflammation of the bladder, and urethritis inflammation of the urethra. Commonly, cystitis and urethritis are caused by a bacterial infection, usually Eschericia coli (E. coli), where the bacterium clings to the wall of the bladder or urethra and causes damage to the lining. The symptoms include an increased desire to urinate, though volume may be minute, a burning sensation, and sometimes pain, on urination, and blood in the urine. There may also be fever associated with these symptoms.

NUTRITIONAL HELP FOR NEPHRITIS, CYSTITIS, AND URETHRITIS

- Plenty of water throughout the infection to flush out the bacterium.

- Cooled boiled water with added lemon juice is very helpful.

- Plenty of vegetables and fruits high in vitamin C—tomatoes, bell peppers, blackcurrants.

- Celery and fennel for (for their healing and antidiuretic action).

- Garlic, cranberries, and unsweetened cranberry juice (for their antibacterial activity).

- Supplements: Vitamins B6, C, and E; zinc; cranberry extract; a probiotic (especially if antibiotics have been taken).

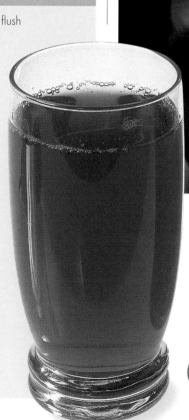

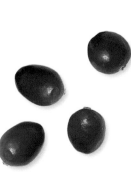

ABOVE **Keeping fit and healthy will help stave off any unwanted infections.**

LEFT Cranberry juice is healing and antiseptic, and helps to ease cystitis.

THE URINARY SYSTEM

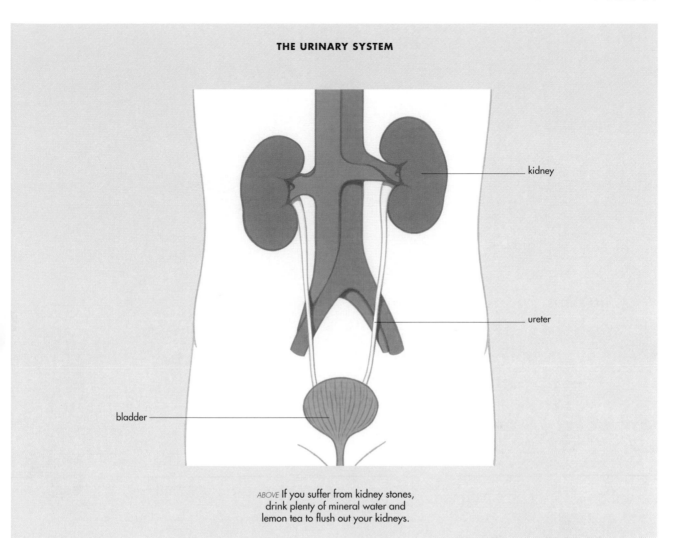

kidney

ureter

bladder

ABOVE **If you suffer from kidney stones, drink plenty of mineral water and lemon tea to flush out your kidneys.**

KIDNEY STONES

Kidney stones form for several reasons, and can be composed of a range of substances including calcium, oxalate, and uric acid. Dietary causes include: excess animal protein and fat, low potassium and magnesium levels, excess sodium chloride (salt), excess dairy food (calcium), sugar, and a diet poor in vegetables and fruit.

BELOW **Kidney stones are painful and are often caused by a poor diet.**

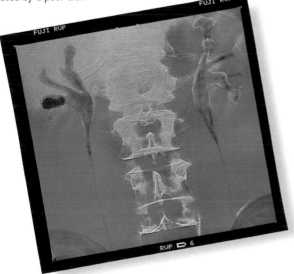

NUTRITIONAL HELP FOR KIDNEY STONES

• [See your physician before embarking upon a program of self-help.]

• For those with oxalate stones, reduce intake of oxalic acid (found in tea, coffee, cocoa, chocolate, beans, Swiss chard, parsley, spinach, rhubarb, beet tops, carrots, celery, cucumbers, grapefruit, kale, and peanuts).

• For those with uric acid stones, reduce intake of high protein foods, especially those of animal origin, including dairy food; have plenty of citrus fruit, and vegetables (for their ability to alkalize the system).

• Plenty of bottled or filtered water between meals, or freshly made lemon tea.

• Have protein from plant sources—lentils, peas, bean curd, green beans, seeds, and nuts.

• Avoid salt, refined carbohydrates, sugar, coffee, alcohol, red meat, and dairy food.

• Supplements: magnesium citrate/potassium citrate complex; vitamin B6; selenium; cranberry extract. *Note: Take care with potassium supplements—take the advice of your practitioner.*

THE CIRCULATORY SYSTEM

The circulatory system is a complicated network of arteries, veins, and capillaries. The main veins empty blood into the heart and the main arteries take blood around the body from the heart. The circulatory system delivers oxygen, nutrients, and hormones to the body's 60 trillion cells, and removes carbon dioxide and wastes from the body.

ABOVE Processed foods should be kept to a minimum.

Many cardiovascular diseases arise from saturated and hydrogenated fats, which block blood vessels and impede blood flow. Fats are also linked to abnormal cholesterol levels—a main determinant for heart disease and stroke. A substance called homocysteine is also a risk factor for heart disease, and can cause clotting, increase free-radical oxidation, and injure blood vessel walls, encouraging deposition of cholesterol and fat. Dietary excesses of sugar and refined carbohydrates can also create plaques and cause inappropriate blood clotting. Lack of essential fatty acids can produce "stiffened" red cells, which are unable to squeeze through fine capillaries. This leads to poor oxygenation of tissues and may cause infarcts in the heart and other organs. Diets high in salt (sodium chloride) and low in potassium can cause fluid retention and other problems leading high blood pressure (hypertension).

Increased capillary fragility occurs when a diet is high in refined and processed food. The red cells can become damaged and the blood anemic if it is not supplied with essential fatty acids, B vitamins, iron, and other micronutrients.

HEART DISEASE AND CIRCULATORY DISORDERS

The common disorders are atherosclerosis, thrombosis, phlebitis, stroke, angina, chilblains, Raynaud's disease, restless leg syndrome, and platelet aggregation.

Fatty deposits form in the coronary arteries, impede blood flow, and cause heart attacks. Strokes occur when a similar process occurs in the cerebral circulation. Contributory factors include lack of exercise, stress, and smoking. Dietary factors encompass: excess saturated and hydrogenated fats; sugar and refined carbohydrates; dairy products; coffee; alcohol. The risk of heart problems is also increased by poor levels of vitamins B3, B5, B6, B12, folic acid, choline and inositol, C and E, magnesium, potassium, chromium, copper, manganese, selenium, silica, and essential fatty acids.

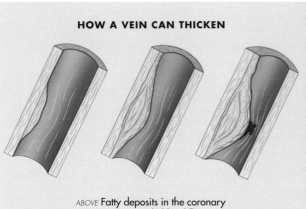

HOW A VEIN CAN THICKEN

ABOVE Fatty deposits in the coronary arteries impede blood flow.

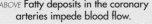

NUTRITIONAL HELP FOR HEART DISEASE AND CIRCULATORY DISORDERS

- Plenty of dark green and orange vegetables and fruits (for their antioxidants).

- Foods to strengthen blood vessels—peas, oats, onion, garlic, fresh wheat germ, sprouted seeds, lecithin granules.

- Freshly ground mixed seeds daily, especially flaxseeds for their essential fatty acids (to reduce inflammation and remove deposits).

- Protein—pulses, bean curd, soy yogurt, seeds, nuts, and oily fish (to reduce amount of saturated fat).

- Whole grains—oats, brown rice, millet, quinoa, buckwheat, etc. (for fiber,

chromium, copper, silica, manganese, and vanadium).

- Avoid dairy food (except live yogurt), salt, coffee, sugar, refined carbohydrates, fatty and processed meats, hydrogenated and trans-fatty acids, and fried foods.

- Two glasses of red wine two or three times a week; cut down on other types of alcohol.

- Supplements: a good multiformula; extra vitamin B6, B12, and folic acid; vitamin C with bioflavonoids; vitamin E (contraindicated if taking anticoagulant medication); calcium and magnesium; high-potency garlic; fish oils; lecithin.

HIGH BLOOD PRESSURE (HYPERTENSION)

Hypertension is often symptomless and occurs when pressure on the arterial walls is above the norm. Dietary factors include: high sodium intake/low potassium; poor intake of essential fatty acids and fiber; a calcium/magnesium imbalance; and excess tea, coffee, sugar, and alcohol.

NUTRITIONAL HELP FOR HIGH BLOOD PRESSURE

• Plenty of pectin-containing foods; apples and carrots.

• Alfalfa sprouts and other sprouted seeds and beans (to lower cholesterol levels).

• Plenty of potassium-rich foods; potatoes, bananas, (to rebalance fluid levels).

• Mixed seeds, daily, including flaxseeds (for essential fatty acids).

• Vanadium-rich foods; buckwheat, parsley, soybeans, oats, seeds.

• Regularly intake of oily fish; reduce amount of red meat.

• Avoid salt, coffee, alcohol, sugar, refined carbohydrates, hydrogenated fats, fried foods, meat, meat products, salt-cured foods, and wholemilk, and cheese, and cream.

• Avoid grapefruit juice if on calcium channel blockers (drugs often used to treat high blood pressure).

• Supplements: vitamin B6; vitamin C with bioflavonoids; beta-carotene; vitamin E (care low dose only); selenium; calcium and magnesium; fish oils; garlic; lecithin.

BELOW A number of dietary factors can contribute to high blood pressure.

ANEMIA

Anemia is caused by abnormal hemoglobin function, which results in poor oxygen-carrying capacity of the blood. The condition is worsened by heavy menstrual flow. Several nutrients are needed for hemoglobin and red cell formation—iron, vitamins B5, B6, B12, folic acid, magnesium, copper, and molybdenum. Characteristic symptoms include: breathlessness; pale skin; dizziness; tiredness; fainting; palpitations. Dietary causes of anemia include: poor mineral absorption; low stomach acid; nutrient deficiencies (iron, vitamins B2, B5, B6, B12, folic acid, C, and E); zinc-induced copper deficiency; excess alcohol. Vegetarians are often low on iron.

NUTRITIONAL HELP FOR ANEMIA

• Organ meats—liver, heart, and kidney—once or twice a week (for iron); no liver if pregnant.

• Plenty of dark green leafy vegetables like spinach, broccoli, cabbage; and dried fruit such as apricots and figs; molasses—all high in iron and other minerals and vitamins.

• A daily serving of freshly ground mixed seeds, especially flaxseeds.

• Wheat germ added to cereals, soups, and stews (for extra iron).

• Avoid foods and drinks which inhibit iron absorption—wheat bran, coffee, tea, alcohol.

• Take care not to store or cook food for too long a time (loss of B vitamins).

• Drink orange juice with egg dishes; the vitamin C will aid absorption of iron in the egg.

• Live yogurt daily; natural bacteria aid absorption of minerals in gut.

• Supplements: a multiformula with good levels of all B vitamins but no iron (iron inhibits absorption of other nutrients), plus separate iron supplements taken at a time distant from the multiformula; extra B12; vitamin C.

THE DIGESTIVE SYSTEM

The digestive system processes everything we eat and drink to supply the body with the energy, building materials, and micronutrients it needs for cell metabolism to enable the body to function, build, repair, and maintain itself. The digestive tract starts at the mouth, through the stomach and small intestine, to the large intestine (colon or bowel), rectum, and anus. Nutritional therapy is concerned greatly with encouraging proper digestion, removing food intolerances, enhancing absorption and assimilation, and encouraging appropriate removal of wastes.

LEFT Drink p
to help kee
your diges
system clea
and in goo
working o

INDIGESTION, HEARTBURN, AND ESOPHAGITIS

There are numerous causes of digestive distress related not only to the food we eat but to the way in which it is eaten. The symptoms often include a dull ache or stabbing pain in the center of the chest, belching, acid reflux, nausea, or a feeling that the food is "stuck" just behind the breastbone. Whatever the trigger, the result is irritation of the digestive lining, possibly because of poor mucous protection.

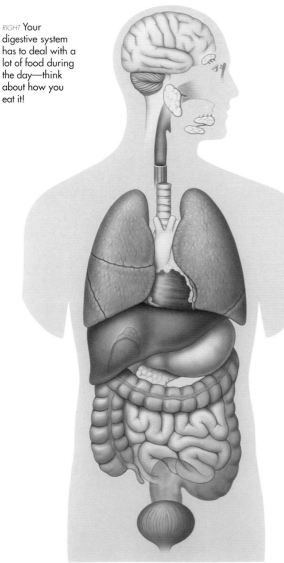

RIGHT Your digestive system has to deal with a lot of food during the day—think about how you eat it!

NUTRITIONAL HELP FOR INDIGESTION, HEARTBURN, AND ESOPHAGITIS

• Eat five or six small meals a day, instead of two or three big meals.

• Drink plenty of bottled or filtered water between meals, but try not to drink anything with meals—this will prevent dilution of digestive secretions and will ensure that food is chewed properly.

• Keep stimulants (tea, coffee, colas, chocolate), sugar, and acidic drinks and foods to a minimum.

• High-zinc foods; fish, seafood, sea vegetables, and pumpkin seeds (zinc helps normalize stomach acid).

• Beta-carotene-rich foods; carrots, sweet potato, apricot, spinach, broccoli (to help strengthen lining tissues).

• Live soy yogurt (for the natural acids and healthy bacteria needed).

• Raw vegetables and sprouted seeds (for their natural enzyme content).

• Avoid eating hurriedly or late at night, foods and beverages that are too hot or too cold, fatty or spicy foods, milk and cheese, refined carbohydrates and sugar, food additives, and common food allergens (wheat, eggs, dairy, citrus).

• Pineapple after meals (for its protein-digesting properties).

• Camomile, ginger, slippery elm, or peppermint teas, instead of tea and coffee.

• Cabbage water—very soothing and healing.

• Try the Hay system ("Food Combining") for a few weeks.

• Supplements: antioxidant formula; vitamin B-complex (especially B6 and B12); vitamin C (as sodium ascorbate if overacid, and ascorbic acid if underacid); zinc; digestive enzymes (care in cases of very severe irritation and ulcers).

ULCERS

Ulcers, whether gastric or duodenal, are an area of exposed, inflamed, digestive lining. They are more common in stressed individuals or those who smoke or drink heavily, and where aspirin-based drugs are used. Poor nutrient levels (especially of vitamin A and zinc) in the tissues are related to ulcer formation. Other causes of ulcers include: food intolerance; low fiber intake; refined carbohydrates and sugar; coffee and tea; strong spices; and excess saturated fat. Recent research has related the presence of ulcers to infection with the bacterium *Helicobacter pylori*, which can colonize within the stomach.

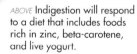

ABOVE Indigestion will respond to a diet that includes foods rich in zinc, beta-carotene, and live yogurt.

NUTRITIONAL HELP FOR ULCERS

• Cellulose and pectins from vegetables and fruits; omit wheat bran.

• Plenty of fresh vegetables, fruit, and freshly ground mixed seeds (intestinal healing).

• Manuka honey and Rooibosh tea, daily (for their antiseptic properties).

• Oregano herb used liberally (for its antibacterial activity).

• Cabbage water (to soothe inflamed areas).

• Garlic (for antioxidant and antimicrobial activity).

• Vitamin A-rich foods; liver, carrots, sweet potato, dark green vegetables.

• Zinc-rich foods; fish, seafood, sea vegetables, pumpkin seeds (for healing and hydrochloric acid).

• Hypoallergenic diet for a few weeks (see page 133).

• Avoid alcohol, tea, coffee (including decaffeinated), strong spices, refined carbohydrates and sugar, common allergenic foods (wheat, dairy, citrus, eggs, yeast), aspirin, and saturated fats.

• Supplements: a multiformula containing good levels of vitamins A, B5, C, and E, calcium, magnesium, and zinc; oregano extract; garlic.

NUTRITIONAL HELP FOR STOMACH UPSET

• While diarrhea and other symptoms persist, have plenty of boiled water; you may also try a little boiled plain white rice, or white bread toasted (no butter or margarine).

• If intolerance is suspected, try a hypoallergenic diet (see page 133).

• Ginger tea (for nausea), or cinnamon tea (for cramps).

• Supplements (during illness)—rehydrating salts (including potassium).

• Supplements (after symptoms have subsided)—a good multiformula, containing zinc (to replace lost nutrients); extra B-complex (especially B12); a probiotic (*Acidophilus* and *Bifidus*).

STOMACH UPSET (NAUSEA, VOMITING, DIARRHEA)

The most common cause of an upset stomach is a bacterial or viral infection of the digestive tract. Food intolerance and dysbiosis are also common causes of nausea and diarrhea which are unrelated to infection. You may need to see a nutritional therapist to locate and isolate the offending foods and increase healthy flora in your gut, or you could try a hypoallergenic diet it the symptoms are mild (see page 133).

LEFT Manuka honey has antibacterial properties and is useful in treating ulcers.

GALL STONES

Gall stones are usually made up of cholesterol and calcium and are more common in overweight individuals and those who eat a fatty diet. Other causes include: excess dietary calcium and refined foods; low fiber; low stomach acid; or food intolerance. Often the disease is symptomless, but pain is commonly felt in the right upper quadrant of the body.

NUTRITIONAL HELP FOR GALL STONES

- Plenty of vegetables, seeds, nuts, and pectin-containing foods—apples, carrots.

- Protein mainly in the form of soy, pulses, seeds, and nuts.

- Slightly diluted freshly squeezed lemon juice taken with the main meal of the day.

- Olive oil and seed oils (sesame, sunflower) on salads (polyunsaturated oils prevent accumulation of saturated fats).

- Ginger tea.

- Whole flaxseeds (1 level dessertspoon) with a large glass of water daily, especially if constipated.

- Hypoallergenic diet for a few weeks (see page 133).

- Avoid saturated fat, refined foods, common food allergens, dairy foods, sugar, eggs, and pork.

- Supplements: magnesium; phosphatidyl choline (lecithin); vitamin C; vitamin E.

CONSTIPATION, HEMORRHOIDS (PILES), AND DIVERTICULITIS

Constipation occurs when there is insufficient fiber or water to enable the proper elimination of feces, or where bowel muscle tone is poor. Chronic constipation can lead to diverticular disease (diverticulitis) and even to bowel cancer. Hemorrhoids are varicose veins in the lower part of the rectum or anus, which become swollen because of increased pressure from compacted feces. They are common in pregnancy and those who are overweight.

NUTRITIONAL HELP FOR CONSTIPATION, HEMORRHOIDS (PILES), AND DIVERTICULITIS

- Plenty of fibrous foods—oats, brown rice, buckwheat, millet, string beans, and raw vegetables and fruit; omit wheat.

- Live yogurt daily (for healthy intestinal bacteria).

- A good color range of fruits and vegetables (for antioxidants and to restore acid/alkaline balance—stored toxins can become very acidic).

- A rounded dessertspoon of whole flaxseeds (or Psyllium husks) with a large glass of water daily

(to help expel wastes).

- Vegetable protein (pulses, seeds, nuts) instead of animal protein; a little oily fish two or three times a week.

- Avoid spicy food, wheat, wheat bran, tea, coffee, red meat, dairy foods, salty foods, refined carbohydrates, and sugar.

- Supplements: vitamins A, folic acid, and C; zinc; a probiotic with fructo-oligosaccharides.

BELOW Coffee can cause digestive problems in some people.

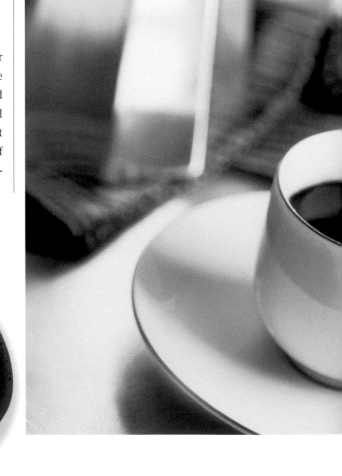

BELOW Apples, which contain pectin, can help with gall stones.

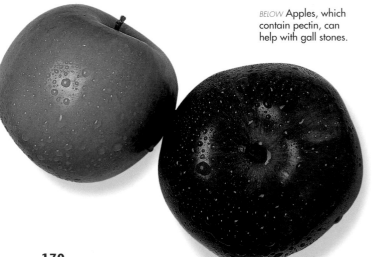

NUTRITIONAL HELP FOR IBS

• Plenty of lightly steamed and raw vegetables and fruit (for their antioxidant, alkalinity, magnesium, potassium, and plant enzymes).

• Plenty of bottled or filtered water between meals.

• Garlic (for its anticandida properties).

• A serving of freshly ground mixed seeds daily, especially pumpkin seeds.

• Soluble fiber from Psyllium-seed husks, oats, vegetables and fruits; avoid harsh fibers such as wheat bran.

• Ginger, slippery elm, peppermint, or cinnamon tea.

• Oily fish, chicken, and plant protein such as bean curd and live soy yogurt.

• Avoid all refined foods, sugar, coffee, spices, salt, fried food, red meat, common food allergens (wheat, dairy foods, eggs, yeast, citrus).

• Supplements: Vitamin B-complex (especially B3 and folic acid); a probiotic like Acidophilus; antioxidant formula; magnesium; zinc; iron; garlic; oregano extract (has antimicrobial action); hydrochloric acid and pepsin (not if ulcers are present).

IRRITABLE BOWEL SYNDROME (IBS)

Irritable bowel syndrome is a collection of disorders sometimes called ulcerative colitis, or spastic colon. It is characterized by alternating bouts of diarrhea and constipation, abdominal pain, and flatulence, though symptoms can be very variable. Candidiasis (or other parasitic infestation) can be an additional complication. IBS can be triggered by stress, food intolerance, nutrient deficiencies, and insufficient suitable dietary fiber.

CROHN'S DISEASE

Crohn's disease produces symptoms of abdominal pain, diarrhea, weight loss, and poor appetite. The symptoms arise because of inflammation (from food intolerances, poor gut flora) which can be very severe, in the large intestine (colon). Nutrient absorption is commonly very poor.

RIGHT Salad vegetables full of healing antioxidants are useful in the treatment of Crohn's disease.

NUTRITIONAL HELP FOR CROHN'S DISEASE

• Plenty of lightly steamed and salad vegetables (for healing antioxidants).

• Non-gluten grains such as rice, quinoa, buckwheat, corn, and millet; minimize intake of oats, rye, and barley, and avoid wheat totally (or try a hypoallergenic diet for a few weeks—see page 133).

• A daily serving of freshly ground seeds, especially flaxseeds, for essential fatty acids (to help the immune system).

• Iron-rich food (to replenish that lost in blood)—liver, dark green leafy vegetables, eggs (taken with orange juice or other juice high in vitamin C to help absorption of iron).

• Ginger, cinnamon, or Rooibosch tea.

• Live plain yogurt; preferably soy (to rebalance gut flora).

• Oily fish, bean curd, lean meat, and eggs.

• Mashed sweet potato and garlic (for the beta-carotene and healing power of garlic).

• Avoid wheat bran and other harsh fibers, dairy food, refined carbohydrates and sugar, coffee, tea, and alcohol.

• Supplements: high-potency antioxidant formula (vitamins A, B3, C, E, and K, selenium and zinc); organic iron

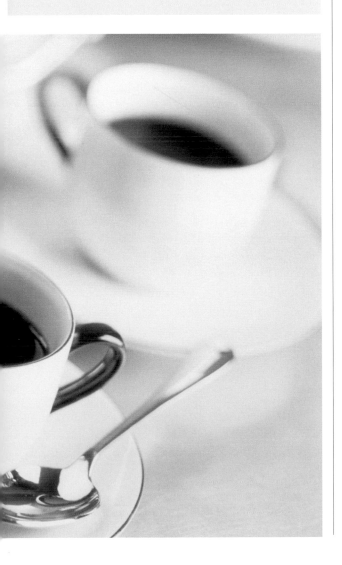

THE HORMONAL SYSTEM

RIGHT Palpitations can be a indication that you are suffering from hyperthyroidism.

Hormones are chemicals that transmit instructions continuously to the body's many systems. They have their effect on "target organs," which may be a specific organ or cells spread throughout the body. Hormones are produced in endocrine glands—pituitary, thyroid, parathyroids, pancreas, adrenals, and gonads (ovaries and testes)—and are released directly into the bloodstream.

The master gland—the pituitary—produces hormones which control the secretions of the other glands. These are the thyroid which produces thyroxine (regulates overall metabolic rate), the parathyroids (regulate calcium metabolism), the pancreas which produces insulin and glucagon (regulate blood glucose levels), the adrenals which produce adrenaline and steroid hormones (involved in stress management, inflammation, and infection), and the gonads which produce sex hormones, estrogen, progesterone, testosterone (for regulation of secondary sexual characteristics, and pregnancy).

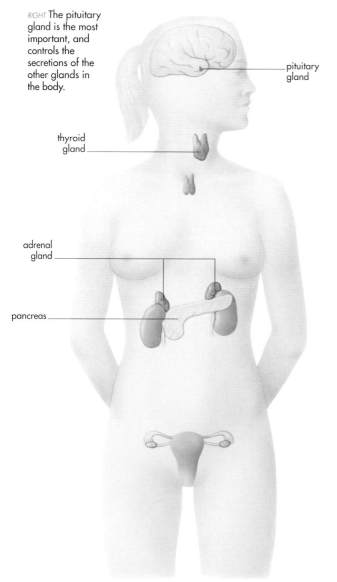

RIGHT The pituitary gland is the most important, and controls the secretions of the other glands in the body.

pituitary gland

thyroid gland

adrenal gland

pancreas

THYROID PROBLEMS

Thyroxine controls the rate of metabolism of the body; an underactive thyroid (hypothyroidism) will slow body processes down, while an overactive gland (hyperthyroidism) causes body reactions to speed up. Symptoms of hypothyroidism include extreme fatigue, slow pulse rate, delayed reflex activity, constipation, weight gain despite reduced appetite, puffiness of skin (particularly around the eyes), and hair loss.

Symptoms of hyperthyroidism include irritability, nervousness, weight loss, digestive problems and diarrhea, and heart palpitations. There are many causes of thyroid imbalance, including stress. Nutritional causes include: food intolerance (cow's milk and wheat proteins particularly); toxic overload; overweight; excess alcohol; fluoride and chloride in tap water; nutrient deficiencies (vitamins A, B6, E, iodine, zinc, and selenium). A wholesome, nutrient-dense diet will enable proper nourishment of the thyroid gland and help hormone production, no matter whether the gland is under- or overactive.

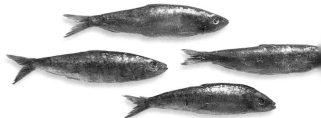

ABOVE Nutrient-rich oily fish will help those who are suffering from problems associated with the thyroid gland.

NUTRITIONAL HELP FOR THYROID PROBLEMS

- Plenty of vegetables, including watercress, radishes, garlic, and edible seaweeds (kelp), and fruit, especially yellow fruits (apricots, mango, peaches, melon).

- Brassicas (broccoli, cabbage, kale) must be cooked; they contain goiterogens in the raw state which will interfere with thyroid activity.

- Manganese-containing foods; nuts, whole grains, and black tea.

- Soy products (bean curd etc.), pulses, fish, seafood, and poultry for protein.

- Oat germ and oatmeal added to cereals (for extra B vitamins).

- A daily serving of freshly ground mixed seeds, especially pumpkin seeds and flaxseeds (for calcium, zinc, magnesium, and essential fatty acids).

- Brazil nuts, one or two a day (for their selenium content).

- Sprouted seeds and beans (for their excellent range of minerals and vitamins and natural enzymes).

- Plenty of bottled or filtered water between meals.

- Avoid all refined foods, food additives, sugar, dairy foods, wheat, alcohol, and unfiltered tap water.

- Supplements: a multiformula (containing beta-carotene, vitamins A, B-complex, C, and E, zinc, copper, iodine, iron, manganese and selenium; kelp (do not take a higher dose than directed).

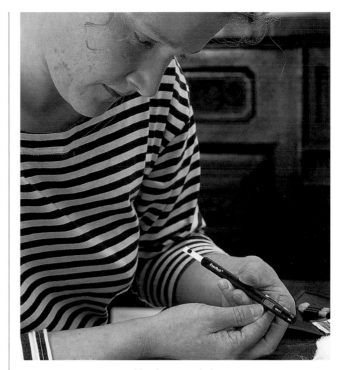

ABOVE **A blood-sugar imbalance may lead to hypoglycemia or diabetes.**

NUTRITIONAL HELP FOR BLOOD SUGAR PROBLEMS

(Diabetics should see a physician before embarking on a self-help program.)

- Plenty of vegetables from a wide color range and including watercress, artichokes, Brussels sprouts, cucumbers, garlic, and avocado.

- Concentrated carbohydrates should be of low to moderate glycemic index (GI), and refined carbohydrates, including sugar and honey, should be totally avoided—eat pulses, rye bread and crispbreads, oats, brown basmati rice, buckwheat, quinoa, and whole-wheat spaghetti as the main carbohydrates.

- High-chromium foods; Brewer's yeast, liver, rye bread.

- Vanadium-containing foods; buckwheat, parsley, soybeans.

- Eat five or six small meals a day (to even out blood-sugar levels).

- Fenugreek infusions (fenugreek is useful for stabilizing blood glucose).

- Sweet fruit, fruit juices, and alcohol to be taken only occasionally.

- Avoid all refined and high GI foods, food additives, common allergenic foods (wheat, dairy food), red meat, and caffeine.

- Supplements: a multiformula (containing good levels of vitamins A, B complex, C, and E, magnesium, chromium, zinc, copper, manganese, and potassium; extra vitamin C; extra vitamin B6 (especially to help with gestational diabetes of pregnancy); evening primrose oil; lecithin; high-potency garlic

BLOOD SUGAR PROBLEMS

The pancreas produces insulin in addition to digestive enzymes. Problems related to blood-sugar imbalance include hypoglycemia and diabetes. Hypoglycemia is caused by an abnormally low level of glucose in the blood and can occur in insulin-dependent diabetics when too much insulin has been taken or too little carbohydrate consumed. Reactive hypoglycemia can occur in almost anyone and is a result of the pancreas overreacting and producing too much insulin. At such times, too much glucose is removed from the blood, creating symptoms of tiredness and hunger. Diabetes mellitus is often caused by the pancreas not producing any insulin.

Recent research has shown that the popular emphasis on high carbohydrate diets may put abnormal stress on the insulin-producing cells of the pancreas causing it to regularly secrete too much insulin, lowering blood-sugar and causing fatigue. Continued high insulin output can cause "insulin resistance," where body cells no longer respond to insulin. These factors may be reasons for the continued rise in obesity despite low-fat diets. To counteract this, foods of a low glycemic index (see page 134) are likely to help the pancreas to recover.

THE REPRODUCTIVE SYSTEM: FEMALE

The ovaries are the true reproductive organs; they are the site of egg storage, maturation, and release, but the uterus, fallopian tubes, vagina, and cervix are all associated structures essential for conception, pregnancy, and childbirth.

RIGHT Oil of evening primrose can relieve PMS.

The female body secretes varying amounts of different hormones, which alter at different stages of life. When a girl reaches puberty, estrogens and progesterone are secreted from the ovaries in a distinct, monthly cycle. Ovarian hormone release is regulated by the pituitary gland via the hormones FSH (follicle stimulating hormone) and LH (leutenising hormone). Hormone secretion changes during pregnancy and eventually tails off, naturally, at the menopause.

Poor nutrition can cause any part of these organs to malfunction. The ovarian tissue can become fibrous and give rise to cysts or, occasionally, ovarian cancer; the cervix can become damaged, leading to abnormal cell growth; the vagina can be colonized by overgrowths of yeasts (see page 162) and bacteria and become infected, itchy, and sore; the Fallopian tubes can become blocked (a main cause of infertility); and endometriosis (growth of the womb lining at sites other than the uterus) may occur. In addition there may be premenstrual, menstrual, and menopausal problems, as well as health conditions related to pregnancy, childbirth, and breastfeeding.

PREMENSTRUAL SYNDROME (PMS)

PMS is widespread, affecting one in three menstruating women. The symptoms can be many and varied; they include radical mood swings, tender breasts, acne, fluid retention, weight gain, cravings and binge eating, insomnia, crying, dizziness, fainting, headaches, palpitations, confusion, lethargy, abdominal bloating, depression, anxiety, fatigue, and, occasionally, suicidal tendencies. The cause of such a wide and debilitating range of symptoms is primarily due to estrogen dominance (low

NUTRITIONAL HELP FOR PMS

- Plenty of vegetables and especially dark green vegetables—watercress, cabbage, and broccoli (for their magnesium content) and fruit (for vitamin C).

- Some raw vegetables and sprouted seeds every day (for fiber and plant enzymes).

- A serving of freshly ground mixed seeds—sunflower, sesame, pumpkin, and flaxseeds (for their essential fatty acids).

- Fish, poultry, pulses, and soy (soy milk, beancurd for their phyto-estrogens) as main sources of protein; have very little red meat.

- Have five or six small meals a day and include a little protein at each one or have a glass of Spirulina powder or granules in water in between meals (to even out blood-sugar).

- Avoid buying and/or storing food wrapped in plastics or polythene.

- Avoid alcohol, refined carbohydrates, sugar, salt, saturated and hydrogenated fats, dairy products, food additives, pesticides in food (buy organic products), unfiltered tap water, and stimulants (tea, coffee, colas).

- Supplements: a multiformula containing good levels of vitamin B-complex (especially B3, B6, and biotin), vitamins C, and E, magnesium, calcium, and all trace elements (especially zinc and chromium); an additional balanced calcium/magnesium complex may be required; evening primrose oil; fish oils; extra vitamin E (where breast tenderness is common).

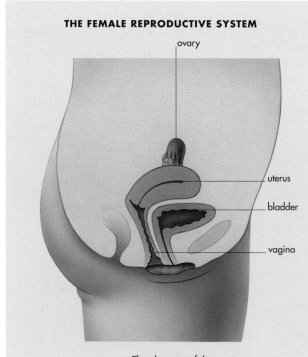

THE FEMALE REPRODUCTIVE SYSTEM

ovary

uterus

bladder

vagina

ABOVE The elements of the female reproductive system.

progesterone) and blood-sugar imbalance, and exacerbated by food intolerances, overconsumption of refined carbohydrates, and nutrient deficiency, particularly involving magnesium, chromium, zinc, B complex, and vitamin E. Environmental estrogens and toxicity are also implicated in the symptoms of PMS, as is a diet with poorly balanced carbohydrate to protein.

MENSTRUAL PROBLEMS

Common problems include amenorrhea (absence of periods), dysmenorrhea (painful periods), menorrhagia (excessive bleeding) and oligomenorrhea (infrequent or scanty menstruation). Sometimes, bleeding between periods occurs and this should always be investigated by your physician. Heavy and/or painful periods may be very severe conditions which interfere with daily life. The causes can include stress, hormone imbalance, fibroids, iron deficiency, protein deficiency, hypoglycemia, and generalized nutrient deficiency.

NUTRITIONAL HELP FOR MENSTRUAL PROBLEMS

• Protein—balance oily fish, liver (avoid if pregnant or planning pregnancy), and lean meat with vegetable proteins such as seeds, nuts, soy, and pulses.

• A wide color range of vegetables and fruit, especially dark green vegetables—broccoli, cabbage (for their antioxidants, iron, and calcium)—and purple fruits such as blackcurrants and bilberries (for their anthocyanidins).

• A serving of freshly ground mixed seeds, especially sesame and pumpkin.

• Avoid refined foods, coffee, salt, sugar and alcohol.

• Supplements: a multiformula containing good levels of all vitamins (especially B3, B6, and B12), calcium, magnesium, manganese, iron, and zinc; lecithin; garlic perles; evening primrose oil; fish oils; protein (amino acid) complex; digestive enzymes.

NUTRITIONAL HELP FOR INFERTILITY

• Plenty of fresh vegetables, especially dark green leafy ones, and fruits (for immune-boosting, antioxidants, and phytochemicals).

• A daily serving of mixed seeds and nuts (for essential fatty acids).

• Vegetable protein—soy, pulses, nuts (for the main protein); a little fish and organic lean meat.

• Wheat germ or oatmeal added to cereals, soups, and casseroles (for extra folic acid).

• Plenty of beta-carotene-rich vegetables and fruit—carrots, sweet potato, apricots.

• Whole grain carbohydrates, but limit intake of carbohydrates in general.

• Avoid red meat, liver, refined carbohydrates and sugar, caffeine, food additives, pesticides (eat organic produce), alcohol, saturated and hydrogenated fat.

• Take care if you decide to detoxify—releasing toxins from your tissues may let them enter the circulation of the fetus should pregnancy occur.

• Supplements: a multiformula containing beta-carotene (not retinol), B vitamins (especially B6, B12, folic acid), vitamin E, manganese, and zinc; evening primrose oil.

INFERTILITY

One of the most common causes of infertility in women is failure to ovulate; it is usually due to hormonal imbalance, excessive exercise, or excessive slimming. Other causes include damaged ovaries, blocked Fallopian tubes, fibroids in the uterus, endometriosis, toxicity, excess animal protein and fat, and incorrect weight (as many overweight women are infertile as those who are underweight). Infertility is associated with deficiencies of vitamins A, B6, B12 and folic acid, C, and E, and zinc.

LEFT Fruit contains antioxidants and phytochemicals.

PREGNANCY-RELATED PROBLEMS

Some problems in pregnancy are serious—pre-eclampsia and Listeria infection. Less serious symptoms arise from hormonal changes, such as nausea and vaginal thrush, and the fetus using up the mother's store of nutrients (for example, calcium). Still others, like stretch marks, constipation, and varicose veins, occur due to the increasing size and weight of the fetus. A good wholefood, low-allergenic, nutrient-dense diet will restore nutrient levels of the mother and ensure there is plenty for the baby.

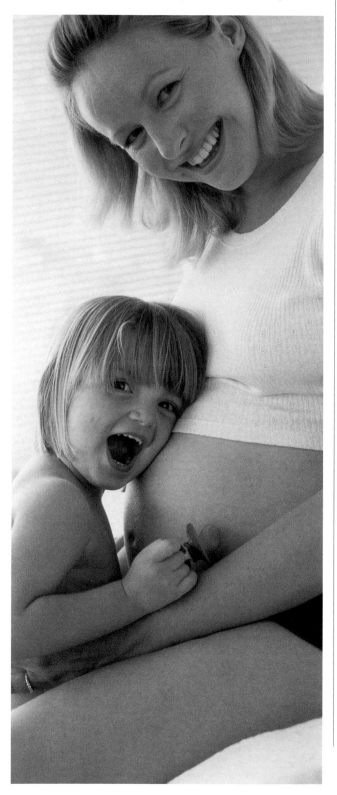

NUTRITIONAL HELP FOR PREGNANCY-RELATED PROBLEMS

• Increase your range of dietary fiber to help prevent constipation—have brown rice, buckwheat, quinoa, oats, fresh raw vegetables and fruit, but not wheat bread or wheat bran.

• A good color mix of vegetables and fruit (for antioxidants and vitamin C)—helps prevent varicose veins.

• A tablespoon of fresh wheat germ on cereals (for extra B vitamins and especially folic acid—to help prevent neural tube disorders; vitamin B6 also helps relieve nausea); these foods also provide vitamin E to help prevent varicose veins and stretch marks, and help prevent miscarriage.

• Cucumbers and millet (for their silica content—to prevent stretch marks).

• Calcium-rich foods—seeds, nuts, dark green leafy vegetables, beans (to prevent cramp)—do not rely too heavily on dairy foods; especially restrict cow's products (allergenic).

• Iron-rich foods like leafy green vegetables, nuts, and seeds will help prevent anemia—do not eat liver, despite its high iron content, since it contains too much retinol.

• Zinc-rich foods like fish and pumpkin seeds (to prevent stretch marks).

• Adequate intake of both animal and plant proteins (for good fetal growth); fish is one of the best proteins—it will supply essential fatty acids for proper development of fetal brain and nervous system.

• Foods high in magnesium—seeds, nuts, pulses—will help prevent nausea; a biscuit and ginger tea, before rising, will also help prevent morning sickness.

• Try to avoid high-allergenic foods—cow's milk and cheese (have goat's or sheep's varieties), peanuts, citrus fruits, wheat—since these may produce intolerances in your baby, even if you show no reaction.

• Tea and coffee—restrict intake; have more fruit/herbal teas and grain coffees plus plenty of bottled or filtered water.

• Avoid alcohol, refined carbohydrates and sugar, processed food, food additives (especially food dyes, monosodium glutamate, aspartame), saturated and hydrogenated fats, soft cheeses (except cottage cheese), and pesticides in food (eat organic produce).

• Supplements: a multiformula (containing vitamins B6, B12, biotin, folic acid, C, and E, calcium, magnesium, iron, selenium, and zinc, but no retinol); evening primrose oil. *Note: Single vitamin B6 supplements must not be taken during pregnancy (see your family physician before taking supplements).*

LEFT Pregnancy is an exciting time, and can be made even more wonderful by eating well.

NUTRITIONAL HELP FOR MENOPAUSE

- Plenty of fresh vegetables and fruit.

- Foods high in phyto-estrogens—soy, fennel, flaxseeds, pulses—help prevent night sweats and hot flushes.

- Wheatgerm or oatmeal added to cereals, soups, etc. (for extra B vitamins).

- Cold-pressed virgin olive oil (for extra vitamin E – vitamin E helps with breast tenderness and lumpiness).

- Plenty of bottled or filtered water between meals (to flush out toxins).

- Oily fish, shellfish, and lean meat; avoid red meat.

- Have plant protein with some meals, like nuts, seeds, pulses (legumes), and especially soy (tofu, etc.) (to ensure low tissue acidity while maximizing phyto-estrogen intake).

- Fruit, herbal, and Rooibosch tea instead of tea and coffee.

- Have a glass or two of good red wine once or twice a week.

- Avoid refined carbohydrates and sugar, processed foods, saturated and hydrogenated fats, environmental pollutants/estrogens (eat organic produce).

- Supplements: vitamins A, B-complex (especially B5 and B6), C, and E; a multimineral (calcium, magnesium, zinc, iodine, selenium, boron,); evening primrose oil; fish oils; (a vitamin E capsule can be placed inside the vagina to prevent dryness).

- Herbal complexes for the menopause—several types are available—ask at your health food store; many menopausal women are using these instead of HRT.

MENOPAUSE

The menopause can produce many uncomfortable physical and emotional symptoms—hot flushes, headaches, night sweats, fatigue, vaginal dryness, mood swings, irritability, depression—mostly caused by the decline in estrogen and progesterone.

BELOW Japanese women have a high dietary intake of essential fatty acids and phytochemicals, and escape many of the unpleasant effects of the menopause.

However, in a healthy women, the adrenal glands and adipose tissue (fatty layer) will continue to make some estrogen, so that symptoms will be fewer and youthful femininity retained for longer. A diet low in allergenic foods, refined carbohydrates and sugar, and stimulants (tea, coffee, colas, chocolate), but high in nutrients is very helpful. Japanese women, with their high dietary intake of fish and soy, seem to escape much of the misery of the menopause; these foods supply essential fatty acids (fish) and phyto-estrogens (soy).

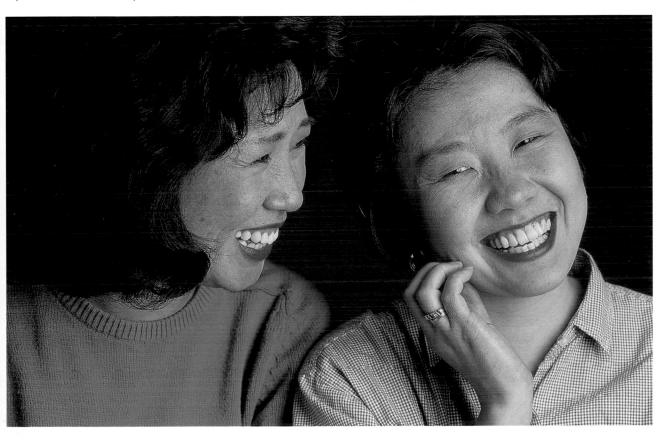

THE REPRODUCTIVE SYSTEM: MALE

The male reproductive organs are the testes, since this is where the sperm are produced; these lie within the scrotal sack (scrotum) outside the body, because healthy sperm development requires a slightly lower temperature than that of the body. Associated structures needed for sperm development, nourishment, maturation, and delivery to the outside are the prostate gland and vas deferens (inside the body in the lower abdomen), and penis.

In men, the urethra, from bladder to tip of the penis, transports both seminal fluid and urine. Male reproductive problems are mostly focused around the ability to initiate and maintain an erection. Much erectile dysfunction stems from stress and overwork and as a symptom of other conditions (for example, diabetes) or medication for conditions (for example, treatment for high blood pressure), but where it originates in poor circulation, hormonal imbalance, or overuse of alcohol and caffeine, a wholesome, nutrient-dense diet has much to offer.

Men seem particularly disinterested when nutrition is mentioned. However, since fairly moderate changes to the diet can make quite significant improvements to sexual function, it seems a pity to ignore the opportunity!

PROSTATE ENLARGEMENT AND PROSTATITIS

The prostate is a small gland surrounding the urethra at its junction with the bladder. Enlarged prostate (benign prostatic hypertrophy), is a nonmalignant growth that obstructs the flow of urine. Prostatitis is inflammation of the prostate gland and often occurs after a urinary tract infection. Symptoms of both include a frequent urge to urinate, difficulty in urinating, and pain around the base of the penis. Nutritional causes include: toxic overload; excess alcohol and caffeine; low intake of antioxidants; excess saturated and hydrogenated fats; excess refined foods and sugar; low fiber intake; cadmium toxicity (from tobacco smoke); and nutritional deficiencies (zinc, essential fatty acids).

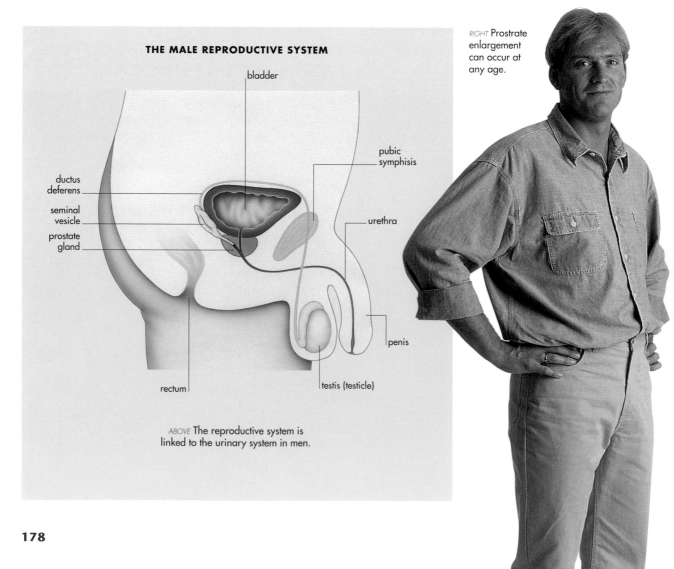

RIGHT **Prostrate enlargement can occur at any age.**

THE MALE REPRODUCTIVE SYSTEM

- bladder
- pubic symphisis
- ductus deferens
- seminal vesicle
- prostate gland
- urethra
- rectum
- testis (testicle)
- penis

ABOVE **The reproductive system is linked to the urinary system in men.**

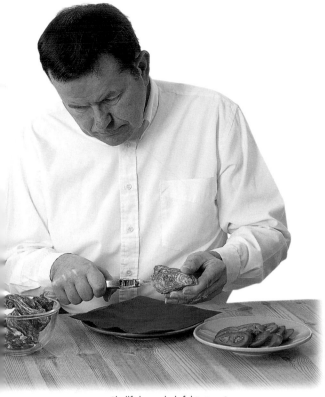

ABOVE Shellfish are helpful in treating prostate enlargement and prostatitis.

NUTRITIONAL HELP FOR IMPOTENCE

- A wide color range of fruits and vegetables (for their antioxidants).

- Whole grains and raw vegetables (for a range of fiber types).

- A daily serving of freshly ground mixed seeds, especially pumpkin seeds (for essential fatty acids).

- Oily fish, shellfish, occasional egg, soy, and pulses as main proteins.

- Reduce intake of dairy foods and alcohol.

- Avoid sugar, processed food, saturated and hydrogenated fats.

- Supplements: a high-potency vitamin B-complex with good levels of B3, B5 (for stress), and B6; zinc; molybdenum; selenium; fish oils; high-potency garlic.

INFERTILITY

Male infertility may account for around one third of conceptual problems. Research has shown that many nutrients are involved in sperm production, maturation, and motility, but zinc deficiency still takes pride of place, being implicated in zero or reduced sperm counts and low sex drive (libido). Other nutritional considerations include: low intake or poor absorption of many nutrients; toxic overload; excess refined carbohydrates; food additives; and excess alcohol.

NUTRITIONAL HELP FOR INFERTILITY

- A wide range of vegetables and fruit, eating at least some of them raw.

- Plenty of bottled or filtered water (to flush out toxins).

- A daily serving of mixed seeds and nuts.

- Sprouted seeds, such as alfalfa, daily (for a whole range of nutrients and enzymes).

- Reduce caffeine intake and have fruit and herbal teas, and grain coffees.

- Avoid refined carbohydrates, additives, alcohol, fatty meat, pesticides in food (eat organic produce), and hydrogenated oils.

- Supplements: a high-potency multiformula containing good levels of vitamin B-complex (especially B6, B12, folic acid, choline, and inositol), vitamin E, zinc, and selenium; extra vitamin C; amino acid complex (L-arginine, L-carnitine).

BELOW A nutrient-rich diet promotes a healthy reproductive system.

NUTRITIONAL HELP FOR PROSTATE ENLARGEMENT AND PROSTATITIS

- Plenty of antioxidant fruit and vegetables, especially watermelon, guava, and tomato.

- Cellulose and pectin fiber—avoid harsh wheat fiber.

- Oily fish (for essential fatty acids) and shellfish, especially oysters (for zinc).

- A serving of freshly ground mixed seeds, especially pumpkin, and nuts, every day.

- One or two glasses of good red wine two or three times a week (for antioxidants).

- Plenty of bottled or filtered water between meals.

- Herbal and fruit teas and grain coffees to help cut down on caffeine.

- Avoid red meat, full-fat dairy foods, refined carbohydrates, sugar, saturated and hydrogenated fats.

- Supplements: zinc; fish oils; Saw palmetto herbal preparation; amino acid complex (containing glycine, alanine, and glutamic acid) to improve urine flow.

IMPOTENCE

Erectile dysfunction has many causes (see above), but those related to a nutritional cause include: excess alcohol; excess saturated and hydrogenated fats; excess calcium; excess dairy food; refined carbohydrates and sugar; low intake of minerals (especially zinc); excess iodine; and excess weight.

THE NERVOUS SYSTEM

This controls the physical and mental activities of the individual. The senses receive information about the surrounding environment (internal and external) and transmit this to the brain via the nerves and spinal cord. Many nutrient deficiencies have a direct effect on brain and nerve activity, since several are crucial to impulse transmission and muscular contraction.

The brain (cortex and brain stem) sorts through the incoming data and responds as necessary, with nerve transmission occuring in a fraction of a second. The autonomic system has automatic control (involuntary responses) to maintain equilibrium of the internal environment—for example, heartbeat, digestive processes, and breathing. Voluntary responses originate in the brain and the nerves carry the information to the muscles.

DEPRESSION AND ANXIETY

Symptoms of depression include listlessness, insomnia, lack of confidence, and feelings of intense despair. Anxiety, however, produces more physical symptoms like high blood pressure, heart palpitations, and gut contractions; it is more related to disturbances in autonomic control mechanisms, though it can also produce intense fear, causing panic attacks. Nutritional causes of depression and anxiety include deficiencies (some B-complex vitamins, calcium, magnesium, potassium, copper, iron, zinc, and essential fatty acids), excessive use of stimulants (coffee, tea, colas), overindulgence in alcohol, toxic overload, excess sodium and a generally poor intake of nutrients, usually due to a lack of interest in food.

NUTRITIONAL HELP FOR DEPRESSION AND ANXIETY

• Foods high in magnesium and calcium; green leafy vegetables, bean curd, seeds, pulses and nuts (for proper relaxation and contraction of muscles); do not rely too heavily on dairy food, since its high calcium is not suitably balanced with magnesium.

• Food high in B vitamins; poultry, liver, whole grains.

• Potassium-rich foods; potatoes, avocados, bananas.

• Add sea vegetables to soups and stews (for extra minerals).

• A good color range of vegetables and fruit (for antioxidants, particularly vitamin C).

• Foods high in trytophan; eggs, turkey, avocado, bananas, and peanut butter (to encourage proper relaxation and a good night's sleep).

• A daily serving of freshly ground mixed seeds, especially flaxseeds and pumpkin seeds (for essential fatty acids).

• Herbal and fruit teas, and grain coffees instead of too much tea and coffee.

• Plenty of bottled and filtered water, or diluted fruit juices, instead of too many colas.

• Avoid refined foods, sugar, salt, caffeine, and saturated and hydrogenated fats; try to eat organic produce whenever possible.

• Meals need not be complicated or expensive to ensure maximum intake of nutrients.

• Supplements: a B vitamin complex; vitamin C; lecithin; a multiformula (including boron, chromium, and zinc); extra magnesium may be needed temporarily; evening primrose oil; fish oils; St John's Wort for depression; kava kava for anxiety.

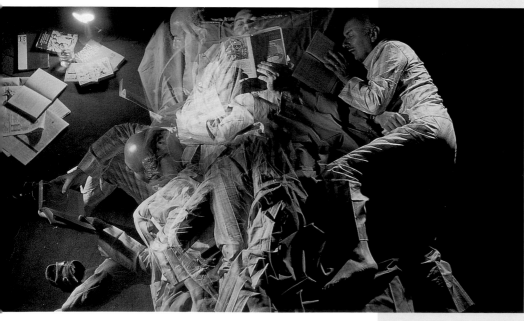

ABOVE Disorders of the nervous system can lead to some very restless nights.

LEFT Ginger tea helps cases of headache and migraine.

HEADACHES AND MIGRAINE

Headaches are a symptom of many illnesses. Causes include stress, tiredness, sinusitis, food intolerances, eye-strain, injury, dehydration, hormonal imbalance, excess alcohol. Migraines are severe throbbing headaches, usually having a particular focus, which are accompanied by aura, nausea, disturbed vision, and vomiting. Sometimes the trigger is a substance called tyramine, found in bananas, chocolate, cheese, wine, and citrus fruits.

Other nutritional causes for both headaches and migraine include low nutrient intake, food intolerances often to "nightshade" foods (—tomato, potato, bell pepper, eggplant), low stomach acid but high tissue acidity, poor levels of digestive enzymes, toxic overload, low intake of fluids, blood-sugar imbalance caused by excess high GI foods, and stimulant beverages.

INSOMNIA

Insomnia occurs when the brain can't switch off; it is often related to stress or depression when there is difficulty getting off to sleep or the person wakes early with their mind racing. Waking during the night can occur when blood-sugar drops suddenly; a light snack at supper time could help, especially of foods high in tryptophan, such as banana. Nutrient deficiencies, especially of the B vitamins and magnesium, can produce insomnia, as can high toxic load. Eating late at night, particularly a large meal, or drinking coffee or alcohol late on, may prevent sleep, since the digestive system is still having to work to process the food. Jet-lag and pain can also keep you awake. Although the after-effects of insomnia are unpleasant, they are not seriously damaging to health, and you will fall asleep eventually.

NUTRITIONAL HELP FOR HEADACHES AND MIGRAINE

- A wide color range of vegetables and fruits (for their alkaline-forming effect and nutrient content).

- Foods high in the B vitamins; whole grains, chicken, fish, beans, peas, nuts.

- Foods high in calcium; bean curd, nuts, seeds.

- Fresh ginger added to stir-fries or chewed during an attack; also ginger tea.

- Fresh feverfew leaves added to salads; or even better, in a sandwich to reduce bitterness.

- Plenty of bottled or filtered water (to prevent dehydration and flush out toxins).

- Herbal and fruit teas and grain coffees, instead of tea and coffee.

- Plenty of low GI carbohydrates; pulses, rye bread and crispbreads, oats, whole-wheat pastas, brown basmati rice.

- If food intolerance is suspected, follow a hypoallergenic diet (see page 133).

- Avoid refined and high GI carbohydrates, common food allergens (including dairy foods) and tyramine-containing foods, alcohol, coffee, and tea.

- Supplements: a multiformula with good levels of all the B vitamins (especially B2, B3, and folic acid; folic acid is a natural analgesic), vitamin D, calcium and magnesium, vitamin C; hydrochloric acid and pepsin; digestive enzymes.

NUTRITIONAL HELP FOR INSOMNIA

- Plenty of vegetables and fruit (to replenish the nutrient levels).

- Eat some vegetables raw together with sprouted seeds (to remove some toxins).

- Plenty of garlic (to stimulate toxin removal further).

- Foods high in B vitamins; whole grains, wheat germ, seeds, poultry.

- Foods high in magnesium; dark green leafy vegetables, wheat germ, whole grains, pulses, seeds, nuts.

- Low/moderate GI carbohydrates, especially at the evening meal (to help blood-sugar).

- A banana or half an avocado an hour before bedtime (for trytophan).

- Avoid eating large meals late at night or drinking caffeine or alcohol towards bedtime.

- Supplements: a B vitamin complex (especially B2, B3, B12, and folic acid); calcium and magnesium (30 minutes before bedtime); vitamin C; zinc; high-potency garlic.

THE MUSCULOSKELETAL SYSTEM

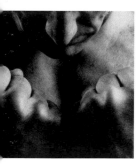

The bones, ligaments, tendons, muscles, and nerves all work together to enable movement, when instructed to do so by the brain. To enable the many bones to articulate with each other correctly and to translate activity into movement, the skeleton has joints which are held in place by ligaments. Muscles pull on the bones via their attached tendons, and cartilage (lining the joints) ensures that everything works smoothly.

LEFT The musculoskeletal system is capable of great strength.

The skeletal tissues bones, ligaments, tendons and cartilage are made up of proteins such as collagen and elastin, plus many minerals (calcium, magnesium, phosphorous, fluoride). The muscles are made up of very specific proteins together with myoglobin (muscle hemoglobin), and need many minerals and vitamins to let them contract and relax properly.

In addition to bone, many other body tissues require calcium to function correctly. When calcium is low in these tissues, it is extracted from the bones and may lead to osteoporosis. Conversely, when calcium is in excess (either because of a true excess, excess vitamin D, or because of insufficient magnesium), it can be deposited in inappropriate places—arteries, liver, kidney, muscles, and joints. Diets low in essential minerals and vitamins, especially if they are also highly acid-forming (as when high in animal products and low in vegetables and fruit), are likely to produce joint and bone problems such as arthritis and osteoporosis. Poor nutrient levels causes weak muscle contraction, and proper muscle relaxation is prevented, producing cramps. Extended deprivation of nutrients may cause muscle wastage.

LEFT Drink a selection of diluted vegetable juices instead of acidic fruit juices.

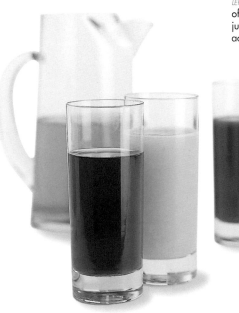

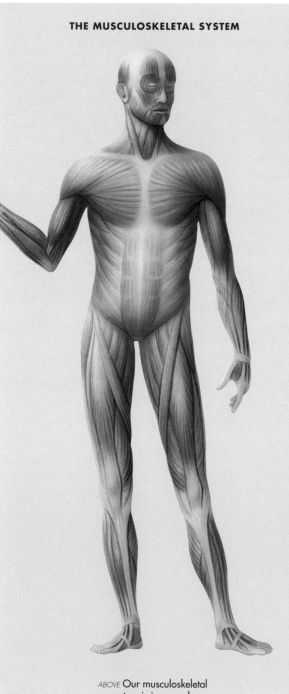

THE MUSCULOSKELETAL SYSTEM

ABOVE Our musculoskeletal system is immensely complex, and maintenance is essential.

ARTHRITIS

Osteoarthritis is a degenerative disorder of the joints (commonly hips, knees, and spine). The cartilage layer is damaged, the underlying bone distorts and the joints become painful, swollen, and stiff. Rheumatoid arthritis is a condition affecting the synovial membrane surrounding joints, which becomes inflamed and swollen and results in stiffness and pain. It may also involve some mineralization of tendon and muscle, making these tissues stiff and ineffectual. Rheumatoid arthritis is more common in women than in men, and usually occurs in the small joints of the hands and feet, but can also affect wrists, knees, or ankles. Nutritional causes of arthritis include excess red meat and dairy foods, saturated fat, excess intake of calcium and/or vitamin D-rich foods, excess salt and pickled foods, high body acidity, refined carbohydrates and sugar, food additives, food intolerance (citrus, strawberries, and "nightshade foods"—tomato, potato, bell peppers, eggplant), gut dysbiosis (imbalance of bacterial flora), and excess weight.

Food intolerance seems to play a large part in arthritic conditions. Pain relief has been achieved by the use of a hypoallergenic diet, particularly when used in conjunction with beverages such as organic cider vinegar; this increases stomach acid and enables better digestion.

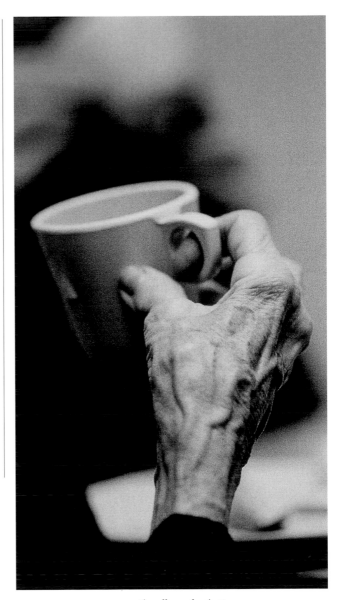

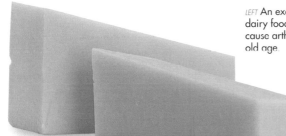

LEFT An excess of dairy foods might cause arthritis in old age.

ABOVE The effects of arthritis on a person are instantly recognizable.

NUTRITIONAL HELP FOR ARTHRITIS

- Eat mainly a vegetarian diet with plenty of whole grains, pulses, seeds, nuts, vegetables, and a little oily fish three or four times a week.

- A good color mix of vegetables and fruits (for restoring alkaline/acid balance, and for potassium and antioxidants); include garlic (for its germanium and antioxidant content).

- Have most vegetables raw or lightly cooked (steamed or stir-fried in a good olive oil).

- Artichokes are very good for arthritic conditions.

- Diluted vegetable juices: for example carrot and celery, or watercress, celery, and parsley (to flush out toxins); also diluted cider vinegar.

- Herbal teas, Rooibosch tea, and grain coffees instead of tea and coffee.

- Soy milk or rice milk instead of cow's milk.

- A serving of freshly ground mixed seeds daily, including flaxseeds.

- Avoid nightshade foods (potato, tomato, bell peppers, and eggplant), dairy foods, saturated and hydrogenated fats, refined carbohydrates and sugar, wheat, red meat, salty or pickled foods, food additives, acid fruits (citrus fruits and some berries), fried foods (except stir-fried), soft drinks, and strong alcohol like spirits.

- Supplements: a high-potency antioxidant formula, with selenium; extra vitamin C; vitamins B3, B5, E, and K; a mineral complex formula with good levels of magnesium as well as calcium, iron, boron, manganese, zinc, and copper; fish oils.

OSTEOPOROSIS

Bone mass is lost gradually in osteoporosis. It is an insidious process that usually takes many years before the first symptoms are found. Often a fall or other bone injury occurs and osteoporosis is found upon examination. It is thought that lifestyle during the early to late twenties is the best determinant of good bone strength in later years. The best positive factors are regular weight-bearing exercise (brisk walking and running) and good nutrition, while negative factors include a sedentary lifestyle, smoking, and drinking to excess. Women athletes who exercise strenuously enough to prevent menstruation, and those women who have an early menopause, are likely ulti-

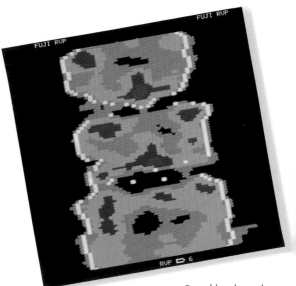

ABOVE Deep blue shows the densest bone and green the least dense in this case of spinal osteoporosis.

mately to have poor bone density. More women than men are generally affected in any case, particularly at menopause, because of hormonal changes (estrogen helps maintain bone density).

Nutritional considerations include poor intake of many minerals (including calcium, magnesium, and boron), high acid diets (excess protein and sugary foods, and poor intake of vegetables and fruit), high intake of phosphorous (meat, soft drinks), low intake of antioxidants, low intake of essential fatty acids, poor mineral absorption, dysbiosis (poor gut flora), refined carbohydrates, salt, excess coffee and alcohol, and excess sodium fluoride in drinking water.

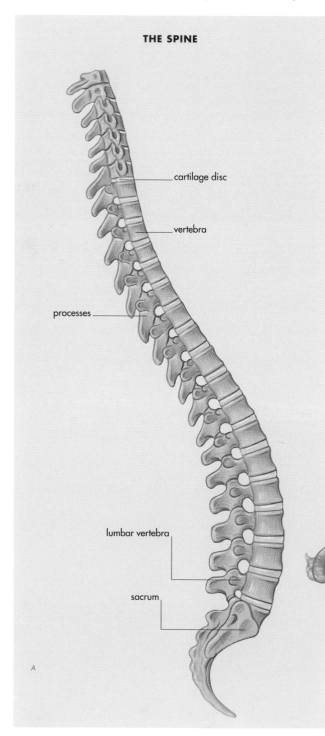

THE SPINE

cartilage disc

vertebra

processes

lumbar vertebra

sacrum

A

ABOVE **Women are** particularly prone to osteoporosis because of hormonal changes.

NUTRITIONAL HELP FOR OSTEOPOROSIS

• Plenty of fresh vegetables (except nightshade foods) and fruit; have some raw.

• A daily serving of freshly ground mixed seeds, especially sesame and flaxseeds.

• Whole grains (except wheat); brown rice, millet, rye bread, buckwheat, quinoa; reduce drastically refined carbohydrates, breakfast cereals, and sweet foods.

• Sprouted pulses (legumes) and seeds (for their high levels of minerals, vitamins, and plant enzymes).

• Add edible seaweeds to soups and stews (for extra minerals).

• Sip a small glass of diluted cider vinegar or diluted freshly squeezed lemon juice with the largest meal of the day (to help digestive stomach acid).

• A daily serving of live yogurt; preferably soy.

• Fish three or four times a week; also bean curd and pulses as main proteins.

• Plenty of bottled or filtered water between meals.

• Foods high in boron; pears, prunes, pulses, raisins, and apples.

• Avoid animal protein (except fish and yogurt), coffee, soft drinks, alcohol, salt, candy, and fluoride-containing toothpaste.

• Supplements: a high-potency multiformula with good levels of B-complex vitamins (especially B6 and folic acid), vitamins C, D, and E, zinc, copper, iron, boron, silica, molybdenum, manganese, magnesium, and calcium; an extra balanced calcium/magnesium formula; a probiotic (*Acidophilus* and *Bifidobacterium*); digestive enzymes.

LOW BACK PAIN AND SCIATICA

These conditions can be caused by many factors, including injury and damage to the vertebrae and cartilage discs in the spine. However, much can be done to help alleviate the pain and stiffness associated with lower back problems. Correct posture, loss of excess weight, and muscle strengthening exercises will all help. Nutritionally, changes can be made to ensure the collagen and other structural materials remain strong and flexible. Dietary causes of weak connective tissues include poor intake of protein and calcium, low stomach acid, poor intake of vegetables and vitamin C, excess refined carbohydrates, and alcohol.

NUTRITIONAL HELP FOR BACK PAIN AND SCIATICA

• Plenty of vegetables, especially dark green leafy types.

• Vegetables and fruits high in vitamin C; kiwi, blackcurrants, guava, tomatoes.

• Oily fish, soy products (including yogurt), pulses, seeds, and nuts as main proteins.

• A small volume of diluted cider vinegar or fresh lemon juice with the largest meal each day to improve acidity in the stomach (for better absorption of nutrients).

• Calcium-rich foods; bean curd, leafy green vegetables, seeds, soft bones in canned fish.

• Avoid red meat, dairy foods, alcohol, and refined carbohydrate and sugar.

• Supplements: a vitamin B-complex (especially B1); vitamin C with bioflavonoids; a balanced calcium/ magnesium complex (2:1 ratio) with boron; digestive enzymes.

GLOSSARY

AIDS (acquired immune deficiency syndrome): viral infection affecting the immune system

ATP (adenine triphosphate): cellular energy substrate

Collagen: a strong, flexible, inelastic protein found in body tissues

DNA (deoxyribonucleic acid): chromosomal material

FAD (flavine adenine dinucleotide): a substance involved in cell chemistry

Fatty acid: part of the fat molecule

HDL (high density lipoprotein): "good" cholesterol

Hemoglobin: the protein that carries oxygen — found within the red blood cells

Homocysteine: a chemical that builds up in the blood and may cause heart attacks

HRT (hormone replacement therapy): replacing estrogen and/or progesterone; for menopausal women and used in treatment of bone diseases, including osteoporosis

Infarcts: damage caused to areas of the body by deprivation of oxygen

Intracellular: within the cell

Ion: an electrically charged particle, either positive or negative

Kcal (kilocalorie = "cal"): a unit of energy

Krebs cycle: part of the energy releasing process of the cell

LDL (low density lipoprotein): a risk factor in heart disease when levels are raised

Lytic cycle: the infective cycle of virus replication

Melanin: the pigment material of the skin

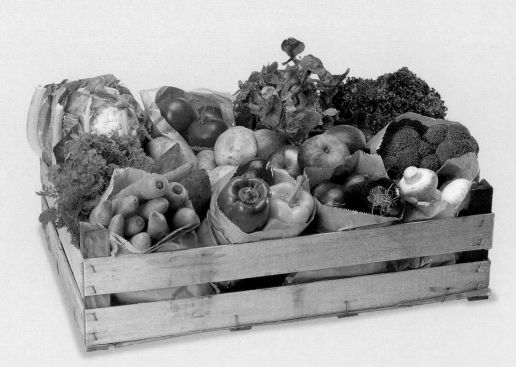

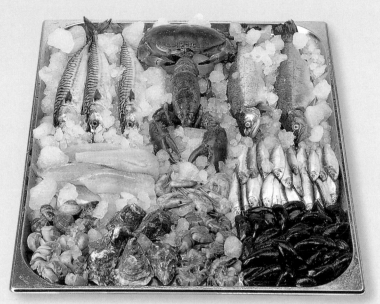

Melatonin: a hormone involved in sleep patterns

Methyl donors: natural chemicals that donate methyl groups to other chemicals

MUFAs (monounsaturated fatty acids): fatty acids having one double bond in their chain structure

NAD (nicotinamide adenine dinucleotide): a chemical involved in cell chemistry

NADP (nicotinamide adenine dinucleotide phosphate): a chemical involved in cell chemistry

Neurotransmitters: natural chemicals that are produced at nerve cell junctions to enable carriage of nervous impulses

Nightshade foods: tomatoes, potatoes, sweet bell peppers, chili peppers, eggplants, and tobacco

Oxidation: chemical reaction involving oxygen

PMS (premenstrual syndrome): a collection of symptoms occurring at regular times in the menstrual cycle

Prostaglandins: hormone-like substances that affect processes locally

PUFAs (polyunsaturated fatty acids): fatty acids having two or more double bonds in their chain structure

RDA (recommended daily amount; recommended dietary amount; recommended daily allowance): suggested level of nutrients required by the average person

RNA (ribonucleic acid): a substance similar to DNA and involved in the genetic process

RNI (reference nutrient intake): an amount of protein, vitamin, or mineral that is enough, or more than enough, for about 97% of people in a group

Tetany: muscle spasm

Tri-iodothyronine: one of the thyroid hormones

FURTHER READING

Adams, Ruth, *The Complete Home Guide to All the Vitamins*, Larchmont Books, 1972

Balch, James F., MD, and Phyllis, A., *Prescription for Nutritional Healing*, Avery Publishing Group Inc., 2000

Bruning, Nancy Pauline, *The Natural Health Guide to Antioxidants: Using Vitamins and Other Supplements to Fight Disease, Boost Immunity, and Maintain Optimal Health*, Bantam Books, 1994

Bryce-Smith, Derek, and Liz Hodgkinson, *The Zinc Solution*, Arrow Books, 1987

Carper, Jean, *Food: Your Miracle Medicine*, Simon & Schuster, 1993

Davis, Stephen, and Alan Stewart, *Nutritional Medicine*, Pan Books, 1987

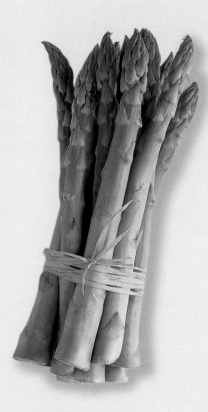

Ebon, Martin, *Which Vitamins Do You Need?*, Bantam Books, 1974

Erdmann, Robert, and Meirion Jones, *The Amino Revolution*, Century 1987

Feinstein, Alice (ed.)., *Prevention's Healing with Vitamins: The Most Effective Vitamin and Mineral Treatments for Everyday Health Problems and Serious Disease*, Rodale Press, 1998

Hendler, Sheldon Saul, MD, PhD, *The Physician's Vitamin and Mineral Encyclopedia*, Simon & Schuster, 1995

Kenton, Leslie and Susannah, *Raw Energy*, Arrow Books, 1991

Lazarides, Linda, *The Nutritional Health Bible*, Thorsons, 1997

Lieberman, Shari, and Bruning, Nancy Pauline, *The Real Vitamin and Mineral Book: Using Supplements for Optimum Health*, Avery, 1997

Lowe, Carl, *The Complete Vitamin Book*, Berkley, 1994

Matthews, Katy, and Giller, Robert M., *Natural Prescriptions: Dr Giller's Natural Treatments and Vitamin Therapies for More than 100 Common Ailments*, Ballantine Books, 1995

Mindell, Earl, *The Vitamin Bible*, Arrow, 1993

Mortimore, Denise, *The Complete Illustrated Guide to Nutritional Healing*, Element Books, 1998

Rodale, J.I., *Minerals for Health*, Rodale Books, 1976

Rosenbaum, Dr. Michael E., and Bosco, Dominic, *The Super Supplements Bible*, Thorsons, 1998

Rosenberg, Harold, and A.N. Feldzman, *Physician's Book of Vitamin Therapy: Megavitamins for Health*, Putnam's, 1974

Shaw, Non, *Herbalism: An Illustrated Guide*, Element Books, 1998

Van Straten, Michael, and Griggs, Barbara, *Superfoods*, Dorling Kindersley, 1992

Walji, Hasnain, *The Vitamin Guide: Using Vitamins for Optimum Health*, Element Books, 1992

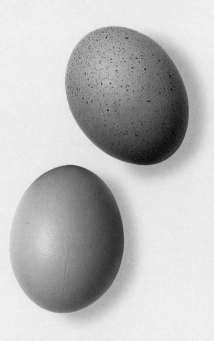

USEFUL ADDRESSES

AUSTRALASIA

Australian College of Nutritional and
Environmental Medicine
13 Hilton Street
Beaumaris
Victoria 3193, Australia
Tel: (+ 61) 9589 6088

Australian Natural Therapists
Association
Taren Point
PO Box 2517
Sydney 2232, Australia
Tel: (+ 61 2) 1800 817 577
Email: ANTA1955@bigpond.com
Website: www.anta.com.au

Association of Natural Therapies
82 Forrest Hill Road
Milford
Auckland, New Zealand

New Zealand Society of Naturopaths
Box 90-170
Auckland, New Zealand
Tel: (+ 64 9) 360 2772
Email: tina@corporate.co.nz
Website: www.naturopath.org.nz

EUROPE

British Association
of Nutritional Therapists
c/o SPNT
PO Box 47
Healthfield
East Sussex TN21 8ZX, UK

British Society for Allergy,
Environmental and
Nutritional Medicine
PO Box 7
Knighton
Powys, LD7 2WF, UK
Tel: (+44) 1547 550 380
Website: www.bsaenm.org.uk

Society for the Promotion
of Nutritional Therapy
PO Box 47
Healthfield
East Sussex TN21 8ZX, UK
Tel: (+44) 1825 872971
Website: http://freespace.virgin.net/
nutrition.therapy/homc.htm

National Institute of
Medical Herbalists
56 Longbrook Street
Exeter
Devon EX4 6AH, UK
Tel: (+44) 1392 426022
Email:nimh@ukexeter.freeserve.co.uk
Website: www.btinternet.com/~nimh

NORTH AMERICA

American Academy of
Environmental Medicine
7701 East Kellogg, Suite 625
Wichita
Kansas 67207, USA
Tel: (+ 1 816) 684 5500
Fax: (+ 1 816) 684 5709
Website: www.aaem.com

American College of
Advancement in Medicine
23121 Verdugo Drive, Suite 204
Laguna Hills
CA 92653, USA
Tel: 174 583 7666
Website: www.acam.org

American Preventive Medical
Association
9912 Georgetown Pike, Suite D-2
PO Box 458, Great Falls
Virginia 22066, USA
Tel: 703 759 0662
Fax: 703 759 6711
Email: apma@healthy.net
Website: www.apma.net

National Institute of Nutrition
Suite 400, 2565 Carling Avenue
Ottawa, Ontario, Canada K1Z 8RI
Tel: (+ 1) 613 235 3355

INDEX